Why Calories
DON'T
COUNT

Why Calories
DON'T
COUNT

HOW WE GOT THE SCIENCE OF
WEIGHT LOSS WRONG

GILES YEO, PhD

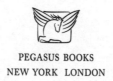

PEGASUS BOOKS

NEW YORK LONDON

WHY CALORIES DON'T COUNT

Pegasus Books, Ltd.
148 West 37th Street, 13th Floor
New York, NY 10018

ISBN: 978-1-64313-827-5

10 9 8 7 6 5 4 3 2 1

Printed in the United States of America
Distributed by Simon & Schuster
www.pegasusbooks.com

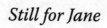

Still for Jane

CONTENTS

INTRODUCTION

I love the song 'Jack and Diane' by John 'Cougar' Mellencamp. This little ditty, released in 1982, wistfully looks backwards at the lost thrill of youth from the reality of adulthood. I say this not to be depressing, nor to imagine some rose-tinted fantasy about halcyon days gone by. I don't know about you, but my thrill of youth was filled with teenage angst and wasted time spent worrying about things that once meant the world, but given the perspective of time, I now know to matter very little at all.

There are, however, two things that many of us do miss about being younger: health and weight. The former, which has been ebbing away, and the latter, which has been gained inexorably over time. The titular Jack and Diane from the song were young and pretty; they played American football and ate chilli dogs outside diners without a thought, and probably managed to stay as skinny as rakes with no effort whatsoever. However, like myself, Jack and Diane are now in their late-forties, and within sight of the half-century mark. All they need to do is look at a doughnut and the weight appears to pile on. They try to work out when they can, but Jack now has a dodgy right knee, and Diane's right elbow is giving her grief. Also, those hangovers just seem to hang on longer than they used to (OK, I admit that this is me projecting here). Crucially, Jack in particular is putting fat on around his stomach area, getting a 'beer belly', and at his forty-year health check-up was told that he had cholesterol levels that were ticking upwards and that he was now at serious risk of developing type 2 diabetes. As for Diane, her blood pressure is a little high, she has a family history of heart disease, and she never managed to lose the 'baby' weight she put on when she was pregnant – and her 'baby' is just about to head off to university! (I'm not necessarily sure this is, narratively, where John Mellencamp was heading with the song, but work with me here, folks.)

Bottom line is, Jack and Diane have been told by their doctor that they both need to try to lose some weight if they want to reduce their risk of disease and increase their chances of a healthy beginning to their next fifty years. They know this, of course; they can look in the mirror. However, between the two of them, they have pretty much tried most of the latest diets going, and the weight has simply been stubborn to shift and even tougher to keep off, not for want of trying.

'Just keep a close eye on your calories to make sure you are eating less, and the weight will come off,' advised their doctor.

'But, doctor, we are doing that! It's so difficult!'

'You just have to try harder. Do you want to live to see your grandkids?'

Ooof. Low blow there.

Many of you would have had a similar conversation, if not with your doctor, then with your partner, or parent, or child, or perhaps a well-meaning (maybe ex) friend.

Just count your calories and the weight will come off. Easy-peasy.

Calorie information is of course ubiquitous. Every item of food that is packaged in any way – raw, cooked, baked, pickled, fermented, cured, dried or frozen – by law has to come with information about the number of calories contained within. Many restaurants, be they sit-down, fast food or take-out, provide the caloric content of their meals on their menus. The same is also true for recipes found in many cookbooks and online. We are conditioned to treat this information as gospel; counting, cutting, intermittently consuming and, if you believe some companies or food gurus out there, magically making them disappear. At times, calories can make us either feel good or bad; or sometimes even good and bad at the same time. Some of us are judged for consuming too many calories, others are judged for consuming too few. We all need calories to live, yet many people feel (or are made by others to feel) guilty about consuming them. While people around the world are dying because they don't get enough calories, many MORE (as of the past few decades at least) are dying because they ingest too many.

Here's the thing that most people have no idea about. ALL of the calorie-counts that you see everywhere today are WRONG.

OK, hold your horses, everyone. Before y'all start @-ing me, which is clearly the thing to do these days, please allow me to clarify. No one out there is actually lying or making up numbers. What I'm talking about is the concept of '**caloric availability**'. The important question to ask is not how many calories are in your food, but rather how many available or usable calories, through digestion and metabolism, will your body be able to extract from this food? It is surprising to many, but the total number of calories in a food is not the same as the number of calories we are able to use, not even close.

Basically:

A – **the number of calories actually in the food ≠ (does not equal)**

B – **the number of calories on the side of the pack ≠ (does not equal)**

C – **the number of usable calories we finally get out of the food**

In the first four chapters of this book, I will unpack the equation above. I will explore 'the calorie', what it is, its history, how it is measured, and where those ubiquitous counts that adorn our food packaging have come from. Next, I'll explain what happens after food enters our mouths; how it is digested and broken into its constituent parts of protein, fat and carbs; and how these are eventually metabolised to generate energy. Then I'll look at what this energy that we have extracted from our food is used for. In the following two chapters, I explain how this principle of caloric availability underpins all of the most successful weight-loss diets, even if not by name (a rose by any other name . . .). The system of caloric availability brings all diet plans under one umbrella, while also helping you to actually understand WHY and HOW different diets work. In the final three chapters, I explore the modern phenomenon of 'ultra-processed' food and its societal implications, as well as how you can begin to leverage caloric availability in your day-to-day life.

Once you understand the elegant simplicity of the calorie equation, you will be able to navigate the supermarket shelves and menus more confidently and begin to look at food, from lentils to a fillet steak to a slice of cake, in a different way. It's my hope that understanding the true science of weight loss will empower you to make healthier food choices.

Every effort has been made to ensure that the information in the book is accurate. The information in this book may not be applicable in each individual case, so it is advised that professional medical advice is obtained for specific health matters and before changing any medication or dosage. Neither the publisher nor author accepts any legal responsibility for any personal injury or other damage or loss arising from the use of the information in this book. In addition, if you are concerned about your diet or exercise regime and wish to change them, you should consult a health practitioner first.

CHAPTER 1

Calories, calories everywhere

The city of San Francisco is actually surprisingly small for an American city, roughly only seven miles north to south and seven miles east to west, located as it is on the tip of a peninsula. To the west stretches the vast openness of the Pacific Ocean, to the north the Golden Gate Bridge crosses over the mile-wide opening to the bay, into Marin County and towards the town of Sausalito, while to the east the Bay Bridge connects to Treasure Island, then to the cities of Oakland and Berkeley in the East Bay. Just a couple of blocks south of the Bay Bridge, on King Street, between 2nd and 3rd, is Oracle Park, which the San Francisco Giants, the city's baseball club, calls home.

I spent many of my formative years in the Bay Area, attending St Ignatius High School in San Francisco's Sunset District and then studying at the University of California at Berkeley. During that time, I became a huge fan of American sports. To this day, American football is still my favourite sport to watch. Living in the UK, as I do now, that means accessing the games via various satellite and online platforms so I can watch my beloved San Francisco 49ers play. American football is brutal and violent, and hence only sixteen games are played in a season. As a result, every game really matters, and the rare times I've attended games in person (it is an expensive business), I am typically riveted to the play on the field.

Baseball is almost the diametric opposite of violence and bru-
tality. In fact, it is only slightly less sedate than cricket (apologies
to cricket fans ... but Test cricket does take five days to play ...
five days!). Baseball, as with cricket, is primarily a summertime
sport, with around 180 games (!!) played in a season. Fewer games
means each one is typically far less expensive to attend, and the
result of each game, particularly those that take place in the hot
and buggy days of midsummer, is less crucial. Yet, a game can last
more than three hours (it's not five days, but three hours is still
pretty long). So what do people do with all that time in the hot
sunshine? Well, there is beer to be consumed of course ... but
there are also many food choices to be made. Throughout much of
the twentieth century, game refreshments would have been limited to the ubiquitous hot-dog, burgers certainly and maybe giant
pretzels with mustard. In the 1980s and 90s, nachos emerged as
the, at the time, height of exotic cuisine (mmmm ... cheese that
stays liquid at room temperature with chopped jalapeños), at least
by the standards of the ballpark.

What a difference it is today, where there are now food choices
galore. At Oracle Park, should the mood take you, there are chichi
wine bars pouring fine Napa and Sonoma vintages, as well as fancy
sit-down establishments with a multitude of plant-based options.
Although, keep in mind this is cosmopolitan San Francisco and
fuelled by Silicon Valley; I'm not so sure you'll find vegan cuisine
at ballparks in less-expensive cities sprinkled throughout middle
America. Even at Oracle Park you are far more likely to find ridiculously pimped-up versions of 'old-school' standard ballpark fare.
For instance, from the El Gigante Nacho Cart you can get Jerk
chicken or beef chilli nachos, not served in a cardboard container,
no no no, but served in a plastic souvenir ballcap, large enough
that, after you've shovelled down the nachos and presumably given
it a wash, you can wear it as an actual hat. Next time you get your
hands on a baseball cap, just turn it over and you will see it can

hold a LOT of nachos. Yet, the US is a big place with many ball-parks in many cities, and this would be considered kindergarten food compared to what is available elsewhere.

If you don't believe me, you can visit a website that breathlessly lists 'The 10 Most Outrageously Unhealthy Foods You Can Eat at Baseball Games Around the Country'.[1] I'm a sucker for such lists. For example, at Kauffman Stadium (or 'The K') in Kansas City (which, by the way, is in *Missouri* and NOT in *Kansas* . . . don't get it wrong like a certain president),[2] where the Royals play, you can get a Pulled Pork Patty Melt. This is BBQ pulled pork, fried onions, oodles of cheese and bacon sandwiched between two pieces of sugar-dusted funnel cake topped with a jalapeño popper (a jalapeño chilli that has been battered and deep-fried). You will note that instead of a normal bun or bread, this heart attack on a plate is served between two funnel cakes, which, for all you non-Americans out there, is kind of a cross between a doughnut and a churro . . . it is basically sweet, deep-fried batter. For dessert, you might want to visit Chase Field in Phoenix, Arizona, where the Diamondbacks play. There you can get a Churro Dog, which is an Oreo cookie-crumb-coated churro (fried batter) in a chocolate-glazed doughnut (ummm . . . more fried batter), topped with frozen yogurt, whipped cream, caramel chocolate sauce, straw-berry sauce (because one sauce is just not enough) and more Oreo crumbs. Oops, I think my pancreas may have just dissolved by simply writing that.

On another website, this one listing 'The Most Insanely Un-healthy Stadium Foods Ever Invented',[3] they even helpfully include calorie information . . . I mean, knowledge is power, I guess? So at PNC Park in Pittsburgh, Pennsylvania, where the Pirates play, you can get a Brunch Burger, which sounds innocent enough, until you realise it is a beef burger, with bacon, a fried egg and cheddar cheese between a doughnut with sugar sprinkles. This will set back the bank account of your waistline 900 calories.

Just as an aside, what is up with ballpark food and using fried sugary batter as a bun? What is wrong with a regular bun? Or, if you are feeling in a particularly decadent mood, maybe even a brioche bun?

At the Great American Ballpark in Cincinnati, Ohio, where the Reds play, you can get yourself a Meat-lover's Hotdog. Once again, don't be fooled by the innocent-sounding name, because what you get is a quarter-pound hot dog wrapped in bacon that has been deep-fried (yup, Scotland, we'll take your deep-fried Mars bar and raise you a deep-fried bacon-wrapped sausage) and topped with beef chilli, cheese and fried salami. The calorie-count for this single sandwich? 1400 calories.

Finally, at Nationals Park in Washington DC, where the Nationals play, you can treat yourself to a StrasBurger on game days. This is an eight-pound (!!) burger, with all of the usual burger accoutrements, served with a bucket of French fries and a whole pitcher of soda. A staggering 10,000 calories, folks. Keeping in mind that the recommended daily intake for an average female is 2000 calories a day, and 2500 calories for the average male. OK, I presume this is meant for sharing . . . but still!

As you are wiping the drool off your face, here are a couple of questions for you food voyeurs. First, while clearly none of the foods I have described above are going to make it onto a weight-loss plan any time soon, are any of them actually intrinsically bad for you? And second, does the provision of calorie-counts help inform, in any way, which of the foods are better or worse for you? Is the 1400 calorie Meat-lovers Hotdog worse for you than the Brunch Burger, which only comes in at a slender 900 calories? If you are someone who counts calories, then the answer is, of course, yes! Five hundred calories worse for you, clearly!

But is it though? In reality, how useful is it to know how many calories there are in a given item of food? If there are more calories in one than another, does that mean it is worse for you? Are foods with fewer calories automatically better for you? Are all calories equal?

WHAT IS A CALORIE?

First things first, what is a calorie? Well, in the simplest terms, a calorie is a unit of energy. To be more specific, it is the amount of energy it takes to heat up 1 millilitre of water by 1°C at sea level. But, confusingly, these are almost never the calories we are referring to when we speak about them in relation to food. Rather, the Calories we are talking about when it comes to food begin not with a small 'c', but a big 'C' . . . no, I am not making this up. A big or capital 'C' Calorie is the amount of energy it takes to raise 1 litre of water by 1°C at sea level. Because there are 1000 millilitres in 1 litre, a Calorie can also be referred to as a kilocalorie, or a kcal for short. You will see this used on the packaging of food to indicate calorie-counts; so the nutritional information on a Mars bar, for instance, will say 228kcals. The problem of course is that while in writing this might be clear (although only barely), when one says the word 'calorie' out loud, it doesn't matter whether it is spelt with a small 'c' or a big 'C', it is still pronounced 'calorie'.

Another piece of information that you will notice on the nutritional panel of most packaged food is the number of kJ, or kilojoules. A joule is the amount of energy required to make a mass of 1 kilogram accelerate at a rate of 1 metre per second every second ($1kg\ m/s^{-2}$, otherwise known as 1 Newton, after Isaac Newton) for a distance of 1 metre. What does this actually mean in real terms? Well, at sea level, gravity is accelerating us towards the centre of the Earth at $9.806m/s^{-2}$, which is what gives us our weight; in order to feel the acceleration, we just need to fall off a cliff (please, don't)! Now, if we lift a 1kg weight 1m off the ground, we are, in essence, accelerating 1kg at $9.806ms^{-2}$ in the opposite direction to gravity (otherwise known as 'up'). If accelerating 1kg at $1ms^{-2}$ for 1m = 1 joule, then accelerating 1kg at $9.806ms^{-2}$ for 1m = 9.8 joules. Divide 1kg by 9.8 to find out how much you would be able to lift with 1 joule and you'll find it is 0.102kg, or 102g. So in the real world, 1 joule is the amount of energy it takes to lift 102 grams up 1 metre at sea level, on Earth (all of these numbers would change if we were doing it on, say, Jupiter).

One calorie is equivalent to 4.184 joules (which most people round up to 4.2 joules), and hence 1kcal is equivalent to 4.2kJs. It is, as you can see, quite hideously complicated, which is why people very seldom, if ever, refer to kJs or kcals when it comes to speaking about food. The reality is that in normal everyday parlance, when the word calorie is mentioned, it actually refers to kcal. I am presuming that 'calorie' is just a whole lot easier to say than any of the other options, so it has stuck! For ease and the avoidance of confusion, I will adhere to this convention in this book. Whenever I use the word 'calorie' (as I did in the opening of this chapter), it is to mean the big 'C' Calorie, kilocalorie, kcal, 4200 joules or 4.2 kJs.

CALORIES EVERYWHERE

Calorie information is, of course, not limited to mouth-watering (to me at least, although I could easily leave out the whole 'doughnut as a bun' thing) and eye- (and heart- and liver- and pancreas-) grabbing stadium food. It won't be a surprise to anyone who has ever visited a supermarket in North America, in the UK and in Europe, or in Australasia, that calorie-counts are absolutely everywhere, because nutrition labelling is compulsory on the vast majority of pre-packed foods. This includes dried products, tinned or canned goods, all manner of food in jars, pre-prepared frozen food (like frozen pizza or fish-fingers), fresh frozen food (like meat or fish) and pre-prepared 'ready to heat' refrigerated meals.

Surprisingly, it also includes packaged refrigerated fresh meat, such as whole chicken or a joint of beef for roasting, and always includes the caveat of 'when trimmed of fat'; I for one eat the fat, thank you (don't judge me!). However, if these exact same products are in the 'butcher' section of the supermarket, and hence not wrapped in plastic (although I guarantee you that the vast majority of fresh supermarket meat arrives wrapped in plastic), then suddenly the calories are not listed.

I have provided examples of both UK/EU and US compliant labels below.

UK/EU Compliant labelling

Typical values	per 100 g	per 10g serving
Energy	417kJ	42kJ
	98kcal	10kcal
Fat	0.2g	0.0g
of which saturates	0.0g	0.0g
Carbohydrate	24g	2.4g
of which sugars	23g	2.3g
Fibre	0.8g	0.1g
Protein	0.9g	0.1g
Salt	0.20g	0.02g

UK Compliant 'Front of Pack' labelling

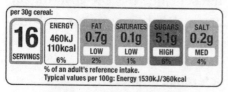

per 30g cereal:

16 SERVINGS

| ENERGY 460kJ 110kcal 6% | FAT 0.7g LOW 2% | SATURATES 0.1g LOW 1% | SUGARS 5.1g HIGH 6% | SALT 0.2g MED 4% |

% of an adult's reference intake.
Typical values per 100g: Energy 1530kJ/360kcal

Each grilled burger (94g) contains

| Energy 924kJ 220kcal | Fat 13g | Saturates 5.9g | Sugars 0.8g | Salt 0.7g |

Typical values (as sold) per 100g: Energy 966kJ / 230kcal

US FDA Compliant labelling

Nutrition Facts

8 servings per container
Serving size   2/3 cup (55g)

Amount per serving
Calories   230

	% Daily Value*
Total Fat 8g	**10%**
Saturated Fat 1g	**5%**
Trans Fat 0g	
Cholesterol 0mg	**0%**
Sodium 160mg	**7%**
Total Carbohydrate 37g	**13%**
Dietary Fiber 4g	**14%**
Total Sugars 12g	
Includes 10g Added Sugars	**20%**
Protein 3g	
Vitamin D 2mcg	10%
Calcium 260mg	20%
Iron 8mg	45%
Potassium 235mg	6%

* The % Daily Value (DV) tells you how much a nutrient in a serving of food contributes to a daily diet. 2,000 calories a day is used for general nutrition advice.

The UK Food Standards Agency (FSA) and the European Commission both state that manufacturers are required to declare energy value, as well as amounts of fat (total, and with saturated fat as an individual value), carbohydrate, sugars, protein and salt, with energy value having to be expressed in both kilojoules (kJ) and kilocalories (kcal).[4] The European Commission even mandates a minimum font size! Although whatever that is, it is still typically too small for my ageing eyes to decipher without the aid of bright lighting or glasses, or both. In addition, the FSA encourages the provision of 'front of pack' labelling, although if included, it then needs to be compliant to certain rules, and while it can complement, it cannot be used as a replacement for the compulsory back-of-pack info. It is used to highlight the apparent 'sins' of the food; calories, fat, sugar and salt. It comes in two flavours – in black and white, where the amount of different sins are simply indicated in kcal, kJ or grams, and in glorious technicolour, where the sins are additionally lit in 'traffic light' signals of green, amber or red, corresponding, in Goldilocks fashion, to low, medium or high 'sin' respectively. Foods will trigger the red signal if any of the components exceeds 25 per cent in 100g or 30 per cent in one 'portion' (depending which is larger) of the daily reference intake. For drinks, the red signal appears if criteria exceed 12.5 per cent in 100ml or 15 per cent in one 'portion' of the daily reference intake. In the published guidance for the scheme,[5] the UK government states that the additional labelling can help consumers 'balance their diet and control their energy intake'.

Front-of-Pack Reference Intakes

Energy (kJ)	8400
Energy (kcal)	2000
Fat	70g
Saturates	20g
Sugars	90g
Salt	6g

What I find odd, though, is that having gone through the trouble of providing detailed guidance (and it is detailed and long) about the dos and don'ts of front-of-pack labelling, they haven't gone just one very tiny step further and made the 'traffic lights' part of the compliance. Whatever you might think of the traffic signals, they are, at the very least, visually effective and easy to understand, particularly on packaging that is often crowded with words, imagery and branding. Many food manufacturers go through the trouble of front-of-pack labelling, but then do it in black and white, which, to my aged eyes at any rate, makes it almost invisible. Might this be a case of a manufacturer wanting to seem transparent – to be seen to be providing as much information as possible to allow their consumers to make an informed decision – yet not give SO much information that they dissuade anyone from making a purchase? We certainly couldn't have flashes of inconvenient red ruining the branding design ... Not that I'm cynical or anything, of course.

The US Food and Drug Administration (FDA) labelling scheme[6] provides much the same information, with a few differences. First, instead of salt, they refer to 'sodium'. Why? Each molecule of table salt is made of one atom of sodium and one atom of chloride, thus its chemical name 'sodium chloride'. However, as chloride has a molecular weight about 50 per cent heavier than sodium, 100g of sodium chloride will be approximately 40g sodium and 60g chloride. So for those of you who travel from Europe/UK to the US or vice versa, it is important to remember that US labels provide for the amount of sodium present (a smaller number), and not of salt (a larger number). So 0.4g of sodium would be equivalent to 1g of salt, for example. But since the vast majority of dietary sodium is derived from salt, the information provided is still an accurate reflection of the amount of salt consumed.

Second, in addition to total fat and the amount of saturated fats, they also include the amount of 'trans fats'. While found naturally in small amounts in animal fat, most of the trans fat consumed today is created by the food industry as a side effect of partially hydrogenating unsaturated vegetable oils. The reasons for partially hydrogenating oils are to increase product shelf life and decrease refrigeration requirements – a magical mix, clearly – and these oils, because they tend to be solid at room temperature, also have the right structure and consistency to replace animal fats such as butter and lard at a lower cost. The issue is, while unsaturated fats, like, for example, olive oil, are typically good for you, or certainly better for you than saturated fats, trans fats have been shown to increase risk of disease, in particular heart disease. Thus the requirement by the FDA to clearly mark how much is present in food. From April 2021 the EU will require all food to contain no more than 2g of industrial trans fat per 100g of total fat.

Third, US labelling requires the amount of 'added sugars' to be separated out from total sugar in the food. Added sugars are sugars and syrups that are added to foods and drink when they are processed or prepared. Naturally occurring sugars such as those in fruit or milk are not added sugars. While chemically indistinguishable, our bodies handle the sugars that are present in whole fruit or vegetables differently from refined sugars. The presence of fibre slows the release of sugar from food, thereby reducing its caloric availability. I will discuss the role of fibre in Chapter 6, later in the book. Finally, the FDA also requires the amount of micronutrients, including vitamins and minerals, to be included.

Then there is the question of how much exactly is 'a serving' or 'a portion'. Some situations are straightforward, such as with individually portioned chocolate bars or small bags of crisps or potato chips. The issue, however, is that most foods are not sold in single-portion packages. Take breakfast cereal as an example. The recommended serving size is 30 grams. Now, unless you are having breakfast at a hotel where they provide individually packed portions, most of us buy cereal in large boxes of 600 grams or more. I serve myself Cheerios in what I consider to be a 'cereal-sized' bowl, and like most, if not all, of you I have absolutely no idea how much I tip in, except that it is almost certainly far more than a 'serving'. I mean, seriously, have you seen what a pitiful amount of cereal 30 grams is? Another example is pasta. For whatever reason, the powers that be have decreed that a serving of dried pasta, whatever your favourite shape might be, is 75 grams. The problem is that pasta, certainly in UK and Europe, is sold in 500-gram packs. I don't know anyone, at least in a domestic situation, who would weigh a 75-gram portion of pasta. I mean, how would that even work with spaghetti? Half of it would end up on the floor! Also, even if you were minded to weigh your pasta, you would rapidly realise that 500 grams divided by 75 grams is 6.66667 . . . so if you were rigidly adhering to the 75-gram portion, you would always have 50 grams leftover from a 500-gram pack. What is that all about? As with the cereal, most of us simply tip in 'enough' pasta, which often means a lot more than 75 grams, because otherwise you would be left with irritating half-finished packs of tagliatelle making your cupboard look messy.

So in practice, the nutritional info for a serving of whatever, including the all-important calorie-count, is next to useless. It is not what most people would eat on a day-to-day basis.

The UK government appears to tacitly acknowledge this and states that:

'Generally accepted portion sizes should be used wherever possible. However, it is recognised that labelling on the basis of a consumption unit, for example a slice of bread in a loaf, is practicable for some foods where a standard portion size varies according to the eating occasion.'[7]

That sounds pretty darn arbitrary to me. First of all, what is a generally accepted portion size? Would that be one slice of pizza, for instance? But many people might often want two slices of pizza. And crucially, what if the 'eating occasion', as is often the case, demands eating the whole damn pack? I require calorie information for the whole damn pack . . . Don't make me do maths under duress!

EATING-OUT CALORIES

Most weekday mornings, I can be found at the coffee vendor on the ground floor of our building, just by the entrance to the diabetes clinic, lining up for my daily caffeine hit. Joining me in the queue will be doctors in scrubs, nurses in the middle of their shift, patients coming in for their early morning appointments and scientists like myself, waiting for their latte or cappuccino or flat-white or Americano. While we are waiting for our coffee to be carefully hand-crafted (or at least that is what the menu-board tells us is happening) and sprinkled with cinnamon or cocoa powder, we are, by design, clearly, simultaneously being tempted by the cakes and pastries on offer. I do have a weakness for muffins (white chocolate and raspberry, blueberry or double Belgian-chocolate chip, in that order of preference), and every morning I rediscover, to my horror, courtesy of a little placard, that a muffin costing £2 will set you back around 400 calories! Eek!

So how about calorie-counts on menus or at point of purchase? Are they also compulsory? Well, that is a far more complicated beast. While a growing number of restaurants and cafes now include this information, it is by no means universal. Since 7 May 2018, the US FDA has required calorie and nutrition information to be made available to consumers, but only in larger chain establishments[8]. The menu-labelling requirements apply to restaurants and other food retailers that are part of a chain with twenty or more locations. In addition, businesses must also provide, upon request, written nutrition information for total calories, total fat, saturated fat, trans fat, cholesterol, sodium, total carbohydrates, sugars, fibre, and protein, together with a statement that '2000 calories a day is used for general nutrition advice, but calorie needs vary'. All of this is consistent with the information that has to be provided on pre-packaged food.

In the UK, voluntary menu labelling was included as part of the government's 2011 'Public Health Responsibility Deal'.[9] So any menu labelling that we currently see in the UK (at time of writing) is still just that, voluntary. Most of the big American chains that trade in the UK, presumably because they are mandated to provide the information in the US, now also provide calorie and other information here in the UK. More recently, the UK government, as part of their childhood-obesity plan, has been consulting on making menu labelling mandatory. In an interview for the *Telegraph* Caroline Cerny, Obesity Health Alliance Lead, said:

'This cannot be a piecemeal, voluntary approach – calorie labelling should be mandatory for all restaurants, cafes and takeaways, with no exemptions, to create a level playing field and ensure people are able to make informed choices about the food they eat, wherever they choose to eat.'[10]

In January 2019, the food-delivery giant Deliveroo who, to those who aren't familiar with their business model, don't produce any food themselves but deliver food for other purveyors, made a significant intervention. They convinced an initial 500 restaurants offering takeaways on their web platform, including most of the big beasts and household names, to provide nutritional information, including calorie-counts, at the point of order. In addition, all 17,000 restaurants that use the portal were urged to follow suit.

The company said it aimed to 'dispel the myth' that takeaways could not be healthy. Will Shu, founder and chief executive officer of Deliveroo, said:

'Deliveroo's outlook is simple: the way to eat healthy is by having more information and more selection.'[11]

Tam Fry, from the National Obesity Forum, said:

'*(Customers) want to know more about what's coming to them and adding calorie labels is a good start. The cynic will argue that Deliveroo is acting before government makes calorie labelling mandatory, but that's immaterial.*'[12]

That may very well be true. However, a poll of more than 2200 British adults, albeit commissioned by the company themselves, found that nearly 54 per cent said yes to the question 'Would you like to see more information on the calorie content of the food you order for delivery from restaurants and takeaways?'[13] So in addition to keeping one eye on the inevitable, there does also appear to be demand, and therefore a cold, hard business case for their manoeuvre.

There has, however, been pushback from the restaurant industry, including, oddly enough, from Deliveroo themselves. They, together with the industry as a whole, are arguing that while larger chains with standardised menus would have no problems providing calorie and other nutritional information (hence the FDA's approach), this would be very difficult indeed for independent businesses, from cafes or pubs to fancy Michelin-star restaurants, where menus often change frequently, sometimes even daily. This is a fair point, I feel, because measuring the calorie content of food is no easy task.

It does beg the question, though, as to how exactly the caloric content of all these food items is measured?

ANTOINE LAVOISIER

Before we can answer the question effectively, we need to first meet the French aristocrat and scientist Antoine Lavoisier. Lavoisier, whose father was a lawyer and mother an heiress to a butchery business, was born into privilege on 26 August 1743 in Paris. Sadly, his mother died when he was only five years old, leaving him a large fortune in the process. While Lavoisier initially followed his father's footsteps, studying and qualifying in law, he eventually turned to science, and is now recognised as one of the fathers of modern chemistry.[14]

Amongst his many achievements, Lavoisier demonstrated that while matter can change its state in a chemical reaction, the total mass of matter at the end of the reaction remains the same as when it started. For example, a piece of wood that is burning might appear to be losing mass as it turns to ashes. Lavoisier showed, however, that if you burnt the wood in a sealed container, capturing all of the released gases and other products, then the total mass remains unchanged. In one of his more remarkable experiments, he managed, by using an enormous magnifying glass to focus the sun's rays, to vaporise a diamond (!!) within a sealed container (clearly when we were kids, and using our puny hand-held magnifying glasses in an attempt to melt our toys or set twigs on fire, we were simply not thinking big enough!). What he found out was that whether the diamond was in solid form or vaporised into a gas, it still weighed the same. He also found out that when charcoal was burnt in a similar fashion, the same gas was produced. From these experiments he concluded that diamond and charcoal were different forms of the same material, which he named 'carbon', and the gas that formed after both were burnt was later realised to be carbon dioxide (CO_2). Lavoisier wrote in his influential textbook *Traité élémentaire de Chimie* (*Elements of Chemistry*) that 'in every operation an equal quantity of matter exists both before and after the operation',[15] defining the law of conservation of mass for the first time.

In addition to carbon, Lavoisier recognised and named a number of other elements, including oxygen and hydrogen. He demonstrated that water was not an element, which it had been thought to be for more than 2000 years, by burning oxygen and hydrogen gas together to form pure liquid H_2O. Hydrogen in fact, to all you classicists, means 'water generator' in Greek. This work eventually played a key role in discarding the ancient concept of the four primal elements, Earth, Wind and Fire (not just the best disco funk band ever), together with Water, and opening up the modern definition of 'element' – substances that could not be decomposed into simpler substances by any known chemical means – and eventually the development of the periodic table of elements.

Lavoisier also discovered something critical that (as with many important and fundamental observations) seems plainly obvious to us today: oxygen was required for the process of burning. In experiments where he subjected certain chemicals, such as phosphorus or sulphur, to combustion, he found they combined with air as they burnt, actually gaining weight during the process. And of course in the remarkable diamond-burning experiment above, he also managed to even combine carbon with air. While Antoine now realised that combustion had to involve air, the composition of air was still a mystery.

In 1774, Lavoisier met with the English 'natural philosopher' Joseph Priestley in Paris. Priestley described to Lavoisier how, when he heated the compound mercury calx (a red powder we now know to be mercury oxide), he collected a gas that caused a candle to burn more vigorously, and that he believed that this 'pure air' enhanced respiration. Lavoisier's curiosity was piqued, and he went on to not only repeat Priestely's experiment with mercury calx (oxide), but also with a number of other metal oxides. Lavoisier eventually concluded that air was formed of at least two components; one part that could combine with metal or other substances, and when released was breathable and could support respiration (forming 21 per cent of air); and another that was not breathable, supporting neither respiration nor combustion (forming 79 per cent of air). Because Lavoisier found that most acids contained this breathable air, he called it *oxygène* (oxygen), from the Greek meaning 'acid generator'. The non-breathable fraction of air we now know to be composed almost entirely of nitrogen gas, with a little dash of carbon dioxide and trace amounts of other more exotic halogen gases.

THE DAWN OF CALORIMETRY

As if burning diamonds, discovering the chemical composition of water and describing oxygen was not enough, Lavoisier made another intellectual leap; he suspected that combustion and respiration were chemically one and the same process. Of course, coming up with a theory or hypothesis is one thing; trying to demonstrate it is another thing entirely. Lavoisier took inspiration for his demonstration attempts from the work of Joseph Black.

In 1761, Joseph Black, a Scottish scientist, introduced the concept of latent heat to the world. Everyone (all living creatures, in fact) is familiar with the concept of direct heat; you touch something hot, it burns your fingers, and you don't do it again any time soon. Latent heat, however, is something that can't be measured with a thermometer. Melting ice, for instance, absorbs a large amount of heat without actually increasing in temperature, staying as it does at 0°C. The same is true during the evaporation of water, a process that also absorbs a huge amount of heat without changing temperature. When the process is reversed and water freezes, or vapour condenses, this 'latent heat' then returns to the environment. Thus latent heat is the heat required to induce a change of state, in water or otherwise, where a solid becomes a liquid or a liquid becomes a gas.

Lavoisier used the principle of latent heat, with the help of his colleague Pierre-Simon Laplace, to develop the first instrument capable of quantitatively measuring the heat given off a living creature, initially a guinea pig.[16] This consisted of a chamber with two outer rigid jackets. The outermost jacket was filled with snow and acted as an insulating layer for the whole contraption, to protect it from changes in the ambient temperature. The inner jacket was then filled with ice, and had a funnel with a tap at the bottom, to let out melting water. The inside chamber contained a hanging basket in which to place the guinea pig, so that no part of the animal actually touched the walls of the chamber, and had plumbing to allow air to be piped in and out and be analysed. As the guinea pig breathed, converting oxygen to carbon dioxide, it also gave off heat, slowly melting the ice in the inner jacket, with the volume of melt-water over time acting as a proxy for the amount of heat given off. Each kilogram of melted ice-water represented the equivalent of 80kcals of heat (the measure of a kcal as a unit of heat was to come later) given off by the animal. With this ingenious contraption, Lavoisier and Laplace measured the amount of carbon dioxide and heat given off by a guinea pig as it breathed. They noted that, in ten hours, the guinea pig melted 0.37kg ice, thus producing the equivalent of 29.6kcal heat (0.37kg x 80kcal heat/kg). Remarkably, they found the amount of heat produced to be comparable to when they burnt enough carbon to produce exactly the same amount of carbon dioxide as had been exhaled by the guinea pig. Lavoisier surmised, pretty accurately, as it turns out, that the food eaten by living creatures was 'burnt' or 'oxidised' by the oxygen being breathed in, resulting in the release of carbon dioxide and heat. Thus Lavoisier concluded that respiration was indeed a form of combustion, very much like a burning candle. Lavoisier called his instrument a 'calorimeter', derived from the Latin word *calor*, for heat (yes, that is also where the gas supplier here in the UK gets its name from) and the Greek word μέτρον (*metron*), for measure.

In 1789, Antoine Lavoisier published his landmark textbook *Traité élémentaire de Chimie* (*Elements of Chemistry*), which arguably launched the modern era of chemistry. Perhaps the most striking feature of the text was its Table of Simple Substances, the first listing of the recently discovered elements. In unfortunate timing for Lavoisier, 1789 also saw the beginning of the French Revolution and the storming of the Bastille. Lavoisier, an aristocrat and nobleman if you recall, complained in 1790 (with the crystal clear 20/20 vision of hindsight, perhaps a tad foolishly) that 'the state of public affairs in France ... has temporarily retarded the progress of science and distracted scientists from the work that is most precious to them.'

A few years later, he was arrested during the so-called *la Terreur* or Reign of Terror, the period following the creation of the First French Republic, when many public executions took place against the background of revolutionary fervour and unfounded accusations of treason. On the morning of 8 May 1794, Antoine Lavoisier was tried and convicted for 'conspiracy against the people of France', and was sent to the guillotine that very afternoon.

Charles Dickens wrote in *A Tale of Two Cities*, 'Liberty, equality, fraternity, or death; - the last, much the easiest to bestow, O Guillotine!'

Indeed. Or as Joseph-Louis Lagrange, the mathematician and a close friend of Antoine Lavoisier's, observed sadly, 'it took them only an instant to cut off that head, and a hundred years may not produce another like it.'[17]

THE BOMB CALORIMETER

It is interesting that throughout his career, while Antoine Lavoisier introduced many new words, terms and concepts, 'the calorie' was not one of them. He got close, I guess, with his papers referring to *calorique* (caloric) and *chaleur* (heat) but never to 'the calorie' as a unit of heat. It wasn't until thirty years later, in 1824, in the journal *Le Producteur*, that French physicist Nicolas Clément became the first person known to define and utilise the Calorie as a unit of heat.[18] His calorie was a big 'C' Calorie, the modern kilocalorie or kcal, and the definition eventually entered the French dictionaries in 1842.

In the intervening years, the use of calorimetry as a research tool, in physics, chemistry, engineering, as well as in the field of human nutrition and metabolism, continued to be developed and improved. Then in 1878, in a military munitions research facility in Paris, the chemist Paul Vieille developed the first 'bomb calorimeter'. While initially designed for measuring the amount of heat that explosives gave off (Paul Vieille would eventually go on to invent modern 'smokeless' gunpowder in 1884), nutritional chemists soon began to realise that they could use it for food. Crucially, as long as they could get the item to combust completely, they could then measure the total amount of calories in any given food.

A 'bomb calorimeter' is about as violent and unsophisticated as its name suggests. You place a small amount of an item of food onto an open capsule in a sealed container, which is highly pressurised with pure oxygen (typically at thirty times the pressure of air at sea level; no prizes for guessing why it is called a 'bomb'). Platinum wires inside the bomb hold the capsule in place and also conduct an electric current for igniting it, burning everything to an absolute crisp; you are literally carbonising the food. Because the 'bomb' is sealed, nothing escapes, and all of the heat given off during the burning process is captured by a surrounding jacket containing a known volume of water. The resulting increase in water temperature in the jacket is then used to calculate the amount of energy or calories contained within the item of food, which is released during the combustion process. Unlike in the ice calorimeter described above, which measures latent heat through how much ice melts, food, when burnt to completion, releases an awful lot of direct heat, and the resulting temperature change can most certainly be measured with a thermometer. And just in case you were wondering, food that is too wet to be burnt, like soup or milk or fruit, for instance, needs to first be desiccated. As water contains no calories, removing it doesn't impact the calorie-count.

So, going back to the question of how the caloric content of food items is measured, the answer is that even today, the bomb calorimeter remains the most accurate method of determining the total caloric content of food.

That being said, and as I mention in the introduction:

A – The number of calories actually in the food ≠
B – The number of calories on the side of the pack ≠
C – The number of usable calories we finally get out of the food

While in this first chapter I have explained how the 'bomb calorimeter' gives us the answer to 'A', it still doesn't explain how we get to 'B'. To do that, we need to meet an American with the most American-sounding of names – Wilbur O. Atwater – and to do that, we need to go to Chapter 2.

CHAPTER 2

The Atwater factor

'We live not upon what we eat, but upon what we digest.'

Wilbur Olin Atwater, 1906, from *Principles of Nutrition and Nutritive Value of Food*

Bottisham is a bustling village about seven miles east of Cambridge, and it was where I lived with my family for more than fifteen years. While the city of Cambridge, with students and academics from all over the world, is relatively cosmopolitan, you don't have to go too far out to find villages where the vast majority of inhabitants are white Caucasian. Bottisham in 2001, the year we moved there, was one of those villages. The 'cultural colour' came from the guys who ran the curry house (previously The Bottisham Tandoori, now Classic Spice) and the couple who ran (and still run) the Chinese/fish and chip takeaway, Jasmine. When we first moved to Bottisham, my wife (Jane) and I really stood out; on one hand because I was the third Chinese person in the village, and on the other because Jane (who is white Caucasian) and I are a mixed-race couple. Just to be clear, it wasn't in any way an unpleasant experience, it was just odd because it seemed that while we knew nobody in the village, everybody appeared to know us! And everyone was so friendly. We would walk down to the corner shop and get greeted multiple times, 'Hi! You must be the new doctors in the village! Welcome!'

Jane and I have PhDs and are not medical doctors, but I'm not sure that this distinction was clear (or mattered) to anyone in the village at the time.

Twenty years on and so much has changed. Cambridge has grown even more cosmopolitan, and this has crept outwards, engulfing Bottisham. Now no one would bat an eyelid if anyone of any range of colour or creed, Filipino healthcare workers, Polish baristas, American air-force personnel or bald Chinese geneticists, walked to the corner shop.

Even though we moved to an adjacent village a few years ago now, I still go back every Friday evening, the one night of the week I don't tend to cook, for either a curry or Chinese takeaway, as I did for the entire fifteen years I lived in Bottisham. I am a man of habit (as Jane will attest to with a heavy sigh) and I order pretty much the same thing each time. From Classic Spice, it will always be a king prawn curry of some description (a jalfrezi or a madras, for example), while from Jasmine it will be a king prawn fooyung (a Chinese omelette dish) and a chicken chow mein. Jane and my son, far more adventurous than me, clearly, actually have different dishes each time (the horror). Oh, and by the way, because these are small independent establishments, they do not provide caloric information on their menus. The routine is for me to place my order, and then during the thirty minutes or so it takes for the food to be prepared, I wander over to the village pub, The Bell, for a drink.

The Bell is a typical small English village pub. Exposed beams, dim lighting, red velvet chairs, with a dartboard at one end of the room. The proprietor is a lady named Donna with a loud shrill voice that easily cuts through the din of a typical Friday evening. And every single Friday without fail, just as I walk in the door, Donna will holler,

''Ello, daarlin'! How are ya! Busy busy?'

To this day, every time this happens, I feel like I'm on the set of a sitcom, with the same regulars sat in their same spots, drinking the same drinks. And I, as a regular on this particular sitcom, always have the same thing as well (yet another heavy sigh from my wife): a pint of lager and a pack of pork scratchings. Now, pork scratchings are, shall we say, not a health food; they are fried pork rinds (don't judge me), and are an English bar-snack staple. They are probably not great for my arteries, nor my teeth, for that matter, crunchy as they are, but boy do they taste good with a cold beer.

On this particular Friday evening, I was in the middle of researching for this book, so I studied the pack closely as I crunched away. There was no front-of-pack labelling that I could see, so I flipped it over and squinted at the typically microscopic text providing the nutritional information on the back. I have to say, given that I was eating fried pig skin with a generous layer of fat (once again, it's not polite to judge), I wasn't particularly hopeful. The energy content for each 70-gram pack was 1832kJ or 440 calories, coming almost entirely from 32.6 grams of fat and 34.2 grams of protein, with a smattering of carbs. Hey, at least I was eating more (ever so slightly) protein than fat!

But as I've said, the listed energy value does not represent the actual number of calories locked up in the food. So where exactly does the 440 calories value on the back of the pack of pork scratchings come from?

'A CALORIE IS A CALORIE'

After the bomb calorimeter was invented in France in 1878, it was German scientists that really pioneered and developed its use in nutritional science. It wasn't, however, human nutrition that drove the science, at least not initially. Rather, it was the nutrition of agricultural animals. This made perfect sense because farmers, then and now, were naturally interested in how much and what to feed animals in order to maximize the resulting quality and quantity of meat.

Max Rubner was one of the key early protagonists research-ing the energetics of metabolism. Rubner attended university in Munich, where he started his career as a young scientist in the lab of the chemist Carl Voit (who was at the time using calori-metry to study animal respiration and nutritional balance), before moving on to become a professor in Marburg.[1] It was Rubner who was mainly responsible for adapting the bomb calorimeter for use in determining the energy content of different foodstuffs, and also for refining methods for measuring mammalian energy output. He was one of the first to define daily energy intake and output in terms of calories. His research centred on what he had termed the 'isodynamic law' of calories: it didn't matter whether a calorie was derived from protein, fat or carbohydrates, it was mutually interchangeable in the body when it came to energy balance. This is often succinctly paraphrased as 'a calorie is a calorie.'[2]

Rubner also built the world's first 'self-recording' whole-body calorimeter. He used it on a dog to show that whatever it ate and breathed in was used to keep the body running, producing, as a consequence, heat and waste, whether solid, liquid or gaseous; like the exhaust coming out the back of a vehicle. Everything that went in = everything that came out, with no loss of energy. Thus Rubner demonstrated that the first law of thermodynamics (that energy can be neither created nor destroyed, just transformed) applied not only to steam engines and other inanimate machines, but to living organisms as well. We will revisit this aspect of Rubner's work in Chapter 4.

Then in 1882, Wilbur O. Atwater, a professor of chemistry from Connecticut in America, visited Voit's laboratory in Munich and conducted postdoctoral studies along with Rubner. Atwater became fascinated by Voit's and Rubner's work on calorimetry, so much so that it ended up changing the trajectory of his entire career, and, as it turns out, how all of us view calories today.[3]

ATWATER AND THE AMERICAN AGRICULTURAL EXPERIMENT STATION MOVEMENT

Wilbur Olin Atwater, the son of William Warren Atwater, a Methodist clergyman, and Eliza Barnes Atwater, was born in Johnsburg, New York on 3 May 1844.[4] He received his bachelor's degree from Wesleyan University, in Middletown, Connecticut in 1865, and obtained his PhD in Agricultural Chemistry from Yale University in 1869. Atwater then spent two years in Germany, in both Leipzig and Berlin, where he was fascinated to be introduced to the concept of the *Landwirtschaftliche Versuchsstationen* or Agricultural Experiment Station. These were scientific institutes specifically set up to improve agriculture and food production. The Leipzig station, for example, was the oldest and the first of its kind. It was set up in 1850 to, amongst other things, investigate conditions of plant growth, such as that of soil and fertilisation; analyse plant feed and its effects on the final animal products; make meteorological observations; cultivate and maintain rare plants; and test new agricultural technology.

Atwater went back to the US in 1871, briefly teaching at universities in Tennessee and Maine, before returning to his alma mater, Wesleyan, to become a professor of chemistry in 1873. It was a position Atwater was to hold for the next thirty-four years, till his death in 1907. Once ensconced back in Connecticut, his experience in Germany continued to be a great influence on his career. In 1875, due in no small part to Atwater's lobbying and persistence, the state of Connecticut set up the first Agricultural Experiment Station in the US, and he was made its first director. During his two-year tenure, Atwater worked on varied projects including, for example, investigating and testing fertiliser.

Interest in the German experiment-station concept spread

rapidly and then the passage by Congress of the Hatch Act of 1877 made possible the establishment of such a station in every state. Atwater was duly appointed the first director of the Office of Experiment Stations, established in the Department of Agriculture, a position he occupied for two years. In addition, the state of Connecticut actually received funding for two stations, the original one that had earlier, in 1877, moved to New Haven, near Yale University, and a new one in Storrs, a small place some forty miles north-east of Wesleyan University. Not that he didn't already have enough to do, but in addition to his national administrative role, Atwater was also made director of the Storrs station; this became his day job, so to speak, and was a position he would keep for the next fourteen years. It was at Storrs that Atwater truly made his mark on nutritional science. Elsie Widdowson, the doyenne of British dietetics and nutrition, wrote in a review in 1955:

'*I think I can safely say that Atwater has contributed more to our knowledge about the assessment of the energy value of human foods than anyone who has ever lived, either before or since his time.*'[5]

Widdowson believed it so strongly that she said it again thirty-one years later, this time in a personal tribute to Atwater that she penned in 1986.[6] The fact of the matter is that Widdowson's statement is still true today, with Atwater's work continuing to influence every single calorie-count that we currently see around us.

ATWATER AND THE BOMB

Atwater's work at Storrs was clearly inspired by his earlier visits to the German Experiment Stations and latterly his time in the lab with Voit and Rubner. He saw the need to provide more information on the composition of American foods, and was convinced that better knowledge about nutrition was critical to ensure the health of the population. He wrote:

'Until about the year 1880, those who wished to know about the chemical composition and nutritive values of food materials were compelled to depend upon analyses of European products, and most of those analyses had been made in German laboratories.'[7]

By the time the Storrs station was set up in 1887, Atwater was already some way into developing bomb calorimetry methods for the analysis of food.

Here's the thing about a bomb calorimeter, though – while it is undoubtedly effective in calculating the gross energy value of a given food, it is, as the name suggests, an extreme environment. The atmosphere within the sealed container where the food is burnt, the eponymous bomb, is pure oxygen pressurised to 30atms or thirty times the pressure of air at sea level. For comparison, your typical car tyres are only pressurized to 2.2atms. The high-pressure oxygen ensures everything burns quickly and to completion, making sure that every single calorie is accounted for. Living beings, however, are not bomb calorimeters. The biological process of food digestion within humans, say, is a little gentler. Apart from a bit of chewing at the very beginning, digestion is, by and large, a series of chemical reactions, accelerated by biological catalysts called enzymes. Don't get me wrong, it is still quite a harsh process – you wouldn't want to stick your hand into your stomach juices, for instance, as they bear an uncanny resemblance to battery acid – but it isn't anything like a bonfire. As a result, depending on its structure and content, how it has been processed, as well as who or what is eating it and performing the actual digestion, each item of food will have a different caloric availability. This is a critically important concept to grasp. *Caloric availability is the amount of calories that can actually be extracted during the process of digestion and metabolism, as opposed to the total number of calories that are locked up in the food.*

If you ate 100 calories of sugar, say, you would extract well over 95 per cent of the energy. Sugar is, after all, our basic unit of fuel. What happens, however, if we eat 100 calories of sweetcorn or corn-on-the-cob? We might well have chewed it and swallowed it, and even given a good go at digesting it, but, if we peeked down as we sat on the loo the next morning, it would be quite obvious that we had absorbed nowhere close to 100 calories of energy from the corn. A large part of it would have passed through us undigested. Consider, though, if the same amount of sweetcorn had instead been desiccated, ground into corn meal, mixed with some water and then made into corn tortillas or cornbread. All of a sudden, a far larger fraction of the energy tied up in those yellow kernels is accessible by the body. Thus, sweetcorn kernels, corn tortillas and cornbread all have very different caloric availabilities, even if we eat 100-calories' worth of each.

This was a concept that both Rubner and Atwater were familiar with. Trying to come up with a method for calculating caloric availability, however, was a far more complicated process. It ended up involving burning loads and loads of food in a bomb calorimeter, and more critically, the careful study and analyses (and often burning) of copious amounts of human pee and poop (ick!), over many years.

Some folks get all the fun jobs. Clearly.

DETERMINING THE CALORIC AVAILABILITY OF FOOD

At the beginning of his landmark publication *Principles of Nutrition and Nutritive Value of Food*, Atwater wrote:

'The chemical substances of which the body is composed are very similar to those of the foods which nourish it. They are made up of

the same chemical elements, and hence the two may be discussed together.[8]

Atwater was, of course, correct, and he considered food to be made up of five different components: water, ash, protein, fat and carbohydrates.

Water makes up the largest component of most living creatures. We humans, for example, are pretty much an assembly of around thirty-seven trillion little bags of water (our cells) that are supplied with a water-based oxygen and nutrient transport system (our blood). However, while water helps keep everything fuelled, in contact and moving about, in and of itself it doesn't provide any calories; it doesn't provide energy.

And how about ash?! What part of us is that? I agree, it does seem an odd term. Here, Atwater is referring to the minerals in our body that, while indispensable to life, yield little or no energy. The calcium in our bones and teeth, for instance, so important for their rigidity; the iron in our blood that is critical for its ability to transport oxygen; or numerous other compounds of sodium, potassium or magnesium that have myriad necessary biological functions. These are the main components of the 'ash' that is left behind at the end of (morbidly) a cremation, or (less morbidly) a combustion run in a bomb calorimeter, hence the name.

The remaining components – protein, fat and carbohydrates – we are certainly familiar with, and they form our main sources of fuel. These are referred to as organic compounds because they are principally found in the living world; in plants, fungi (which are not plants) and animals. They are all composed of differing proportions and configurations of carbon, hydrogen and oxygen, with some also containing nitrogen, phosphorous, sulphur as well as a smattering of other elements.

The approach that Atwater (and Rubner from across the pond) took to determining the caloric availability of food was necessarily systematic and unavoidably laborious. It was split into three stages.

First, there needed to be a comprehensive (as far as it was possible) collation of different 'typical' food items and their composition (water, ash, fat, carbohydrates and protein). Second, the 'heat of combustion' of each of these foods needed to be measured using a bomb calorimeter, producing the gross caloric content for each item. Third, each of these items needed to be fed to a human being, and the resulting waste products from said human, fed said food, needed to be analysed with a fine-tooth comb (not literally . . . well, literally studying human pee and poop, but not literally with a fine-tooth comb). Subtract the caloric content of the waste products from the gross number of calories in the starting material, and you get the caloric availability of the food! Easy-peasy!

Except, of course, that life is always more complicated than anyone really wishes or anticipates. Elsie Widdowson said it best when reviewing the field in 1955:

'The whole subject is very complicated and the attempts which people have made to assess the energy value of human food can only be described as a comedy of errors.'[9]

But I am getting ahead of myself here.

So what did all that figurative fine-tooth combing of poop reveal? After analysing thousands of different food items, Atwater found that in humans, fat, carbs and protein had very different biological availabilities. Atwater called this availability 'metabolisable energy'. On top of that, the specific ratios and how they are combined, whether within a single food item or as part of a broader meal or diet, also influenced the metabolisable energy of the three organic macronutrients.

Fat

Let's start with the least complicated and most energy dense of the three macronutrients, which is fat.

Atwater found that the heat of combustion for animal-derived fat was on average 9.4 calories per gram, and for plant-derived fat 9.3 calories per gram. Why the difference between animals and plants? Because, on average, animal fat is going to be more saturated than plant-based fat. This is why animal fat (fat from fish being the exception) is typically solid at room temperature, whereas plant fats such as vegetable, olive and nut oils stay liquid at room temperature. Crucially, Atwater then found that 5 per cent of animal fat and 10 per cent of plant fat was lost through faecal matter (poop), meaning the metabolisable energy of animal fat was 95 per cent and plant fat was 90 per cent. Put another way, for every 9.4 calories of animal fat eaten, 8.93 calories are absorbed, while for every 9.3 calories of plant fat eaten, 8.37 calories are absorbed.

Amongst the many other different studies performed by Atwater is one where he carefully catalogued and studied the diets of 185 American families over a period of time.[10] One of the interesting things he found was that in the average American diet (assuming that the 185 study families were 'average'), 92 per cent of the fat, 5 per cent of the carbohydrate and 61 per cent of the protein came from animal sources and the remainder from plant sources. The carbohydrate and protein numbers look about right even today. But take a look at fat . . . 92 per cent from animal sources?! Given that most of us don't cook much with lard these days (except on a Sunday when I use goose or duck fat to make my roast potatoes . . . mmmm), but use olive oil, rapeseed oil, sunflower oil or nut oils instead, this seems to be an extraordinarily high number! Regardless, it was probably reflective of the way people ate at the end of the nineteenth century. Thus, Atwater took a weighted average, and settled at a calorically available fuel value of fat at 8.9 calories/gram. This was, very soon after, rounded up (no one ever learnt their 8.9 multiplication tables at school, after all) to 9 calories per gram of fat.

Carbohydrates

Now, what about carbs? One curiosity was that, unlike fat and protein, rather than being analysed directly, the total carbohydrate content of foods was, instead, calculated 'by difference'. This meant that the other constituents in the food (protein, fat, water and ash) were first determined individually, added together and then sub-tracted from the total weight of the food. Hence, this is referred to as 'total carbohydrate by difference' and was the approach used by Atwater.

Atwater found that the heat of combustion for animal-derived carbs was, on average, 3.9 calories per gram, and for plant-derived carbs 4.15 calories per gram. What is an 'animal carb', you might be asking? It is a good question, because animals (humans included) store very little energy in carbohydrate form; perhaps just a little bit of glycogen in the muscles and liver, but only if well fed. However, the term 'carbohydrate' is a broad church, covering everything from simple sugars to starches, to the often-overlooked cellulose and other dietary fibre. So lactose, for example, which is the primary sugar found in milk and other dairy products, would be an animal-based carbohydrate. There are also going to be trace amounts of sugars, in addition to glycogen, in meat. As for plant-derived carbs, that really then does cover a broad range of compounds; we will return to discuss the implications of this later in the book.

With regards to availability, Atwater found that 2 per cent of animal carbs and 3 per cent of plant carbs are lost through faecal matter (98 per cent and 97 per cent metabolisable energy respec-tively). This means that for every 3.9 calories of animal carb eaten, 3.82 calories are absorbed, while for every 4.15 calories of plant carb eaten, 4.03 calories are absorbed. Given that 95 per cent of the carbs that the 'average American family' consumed came from plants, Atwater eventually settled on a metabolisable fuel value of carbs of 4 calories per gram of carbohydrate.

Protein

And finally, that leaves protein, the most chemically complex of the three macronutrients.

We store the vast majority of nutrients that we absorb but don't use immediately as fat, with a small percentage of carbs being stored as glycogen. Fat and carbohydrates are composed entirely of carbon, hydrogen and oxygen, just in differing proportions and configurations. Thus, once they are digested and move across from the gut and into our bloodstream, they undergo only one of two fates: they are either used or they are stored. Except in people with diabetes, who lose sugar through their urine (we will look at how we convert food to energy, and what happens when it goes wrong, in Chapter 3), once fat and carbs are absorbed into your body, there is no magical way of getting rid of the energy; you can't physically wee it out, poop it out, or sweat it out. The ONLY way to get rid of fat or carbs from the body is to use it, to burn it off.

Protein, however, while also composed of a large proportion of the ubiquitous carbon, hydrogen and oxygen, crucially also contains significant amounts of nitrogen. Excluding water and fat, the human body is made up almost entirely of protein. Protein is the main component of muscles, bones, organs, skin, nails . . . any part of us that provides structural support or does any work, essentially. The protein that we eat goes to the maintenance and repair of our organs, and when we are active, maintaining or (when exercising heavily) building muscle. But protein is nearly all functional; we simply don't have a store of unused protein being saved for a rainy day. Instead, any protein that we don't use immediately is (you got it) converted to fat. Crucially, however, because fat is only made from carbon, hydrogen and oxygen, this then leaves a large amount of nitrogen that needs to be removed from the body. Typically the waste nitrogen is converted into urea, uric acid, and creatinine, and then it is excreted in our urine and faeces. Incidentally, this therefore becomes an important component of the 'nitrogen cycle' in the world. While animals get all the nitrogen they need from eating plants and/or other animals, plants get their nitrogen, in part, from animal urine and faeces (and also of course through the 'circle of life', when living beings die and decompose . . . as all parents know, Disney's *The Lion King* is actually a documentary). Thus, in the context of plants, wee and poop act as fertilisers.

There were two big issues that Atwater (and Rubner) had to grapple with when attempting to calculate the metabolisable energy of protein. The first was actually trying to figure out the protein content of different foods to begin with, and the second was working out exactly how much nitrogen was being lost in the wee and poop.

So, problem number one: how to calculate total protein content. While the fat content of food was measured directly, and carbohydrates inferred 'by difference', the protein content of food was, for many years (and surprisingly frequently still today), determined on the basis of total nitrogen content. The amount of nitrogen, in grams, was then multiplied by some factor to arrive at total protein content.

This sounds straightforward enough until you realise that protein is not just some homogenous amorphous lump of stuff. It is now estimated that the human body, for example, contains somewhere between 80,000 to 400,000 different proteins. They aren't all produced throughout the body all of the time, however. Rather, depending on the function of each organ or cell type, different repertoires of proteins are then produced. Each protein is comprised of different proportions of twenty distinct building blocks called 'amino acids' (and for all of you aficionados, yes, I realise there are twenty-two if you count 'atypical' amino acids). Each of these amino acids have different characteristics, such as, for instance, a range of sizes, whether they 'like' water (hydrophilic) or 'dislike' water (hydrophobic), or whether they are (electrically) positively or negatively charged. Each protein, depending on what it is designed to do, and where in the body it resides, is composed of hundreds or thousands of these amino acids in uniquely different combinations, and then origamied into a 3D functional unit to do its intended job. The issue is that each amino acid contains a different percentage of nitrogen. Atwater settled on a figure of 16 per cent, based on the average amino-acid composition of meat; that is, a typical piece of meat would contain 16 per cent nitrogen. To calculate the total amount of protein, you first need to divide 100 per cent by 16 per cent to get a conversion factor of 6.25, then, by taking the nitrogen content in grams, let's say 1 gram, and multiplying it by 6.25, you end up with a total protein amount of 6.25 grams. If all of this sounds suspiciously loosey goosey and a little bit *comme ci, comme ça*, that's because it is! We will revisit these numbers later.

And problem number two: how about all of the nitrogen lost through the wee and poop? As it turns out, far more nitrogen is lost through urine than through faeces. When Atwater evaporated all the water from urine and analysed the resulting dried nitrogenous compounds by bomb calorimeter, he found that the material had a heat of combustion of 7.8 to 7.9 calories per gram. This is approximately equivalent to 1.25 calories per gram of protein eaten (7.8 calories per gram divided by the 6.25 conversion factor) that is lost in the urine. In addition, Atwater found that 3 per cent of animal-based and 15 per cent of plant-based protein was lost through the faeces.

So putting this whole complicated protein section together, Atwater found that the heat of combustion for protein, whether from animal or plant, was 5.65 calories per gram. This means that for every 5.65 calories of animal protein eaten (after subtracting for the losses described above), 4.25 calories are absorbed, while for every 5.65 calories of plant protein eaten, 3.55 calories are absorbed. Given that, at the time of his calculations, 61 per cent of the protein that the 'average American family' consumed came from animals, Atwater eventually settled on a metabolisable fuel value of protein of 4 calories per gram of protein.

THE ATWATER GENERAL FACTOR SYSTEM

Table 1			Available Energy	
Nutrient	Heat of combustion calories/gram	% availability	Available nutrients calories/gram	Total nutrients calories/gram
Fat:				
Animal	9.4	95%	9.4	8.95
Plant	9.3	90%	9.3	8.35
Carbohydrates:				
Animal	3.9	98%	3.9	3.8
Plant	4.15	97%	4.15	4
Protein:				
Animal	5.65	97%	4.4*	4.25†
Plant	5.65	85%	4.4*	3.55†

* Heat of Combustion less 1.25 to allow for loss in urine
† 1.25 deducted after calculation of the fuel value of available protein, e.g. $5.65 \times 0.85 = 4.8$, $4.8 - 1.25 = 3.55$

The Atwater general factors
9 calories (37kJ) per gram for fat
4 calories (17kJ) per gram for carbohydrates
4 calories (17kJ) per gram for protein

As I mentioned previously, Rubner was also undertaking the same task, at around the same time, in Germany. There were, however, two key differences in how he calculated his numbers. First, even though he had the means and was analysing samples for nitrogen loss anyway, Rubner, inexplicably, made no allowance for losses in the faeces when deriving his calorie conversion for fat and carbohydrates. Second, he made the assumption that the average nitrogen content in protein was 15.5 per cent (as opposed to the 16 per cent that Atwater used), which equated to a protein conversion factor of 6.45. It became clear fairly quickly that 6.45 was too high a conversion factor, and he was systematically over-estimating the amount of protein in food. Rubner's proposed factors were 9.3 calories per gram for fat, 4.1 calories per gram for carbohydrates and 4.1 calories per gram for protein. In part because of the caveats discussed above, it was (like the battle between VHS and Betamax . . . and, yes, I am showing my age with that particular analogy) the Atwater factors that stuck.

Thus, the energy values of **9 calories (37kJ) per gram for fat, 4 calories (17kJ) per gram for carbohydrates and 4 calories (17kJ) per gram for protein**, together with alcohol (more about this on page 45), which Atwater found to have an energy value of 7 calories (29kJ) per gram, form the 'Atwater general factor system' (see Table 1), which he initially proposed in 1900.[11] Using these factors, Atwater went on to publish a series of US Department of Agriculture farmers' bulletins, where he catalogued thousands of individual American foods, providing their nutritional composition (water, ash, fat, carbohydrates and protein) and their fuel value in calories. In fact, Atwater was the first to introduce the concept of 'the calorie' as a measure of energy, both in food and in expenditure, to the American public, and these bulletin publications became enormously popular. The separate bulletins were eventually compiled into Atwater's landmark *Principles of Nutrition and Nutritive Value of Food*[12] where, in addition to the widely used food tables, he also wrote about basic nutritional principles as they were understood in the early 1900s. Sadly, Atwater suffered a debilitating stroke in November of 1904, and was no longer able to work. He died in 1907. The book (maybe that is too grand a word for a lean publication of forty-eight pages, in microscopic font; more a compilation, perhaps), which was published in 1906, was actually collated and put together by his daughter, Helen Atwater, a scientist in her own right. *Principles of Nutrition and Nutritive Value of Food* was reprinted in 1910, and then again in 1916 (which is the version that I found available for sale online).

A perusal of the food tables provides an interesting window

into the larders, kitchens and dining-room tables of America in the early 1900s. Under the 'beef' section, in addition to cuts and joints we would recognise today, such as porterhouse, sirloin and rib, are some interesting 'processed' products, such as 'canned boiled beef' (yum . . .) and pickled tongue (double yum . . . actually I quite like beef tongue, I have just never had it pickled). There is also a section on different cuts of veal, which we clearly eat a lot less of today, at least in the UK and the US. The selection of cuts of mutton (meat from a sheep that is older than a year, typically up to three years) is more extensive than that of lamb; I mean, when is the last time you saw mutton on a menu or in the supermarket? Having eaten curried mutton when I was a child in Singapore, I can see that its strong flavour would be a somewhat acquired taste. The vast majority of 'sheep meat' that is consumed today, certainly within the Anglophone world, is now that of the younger and less strongly flavoured lamb. Under the fresh fish section is cod, halibut and mackerel, but interestingly no salmon. Salmon was only available canned, together with sardines, because they had to be line caught during the salmon run in the autumn and were therefore an expensive luxury. Salmon farming only became an industry in Norway in the 1980s, before the method spread across the globe; today, approximately 60 per cent of the world's salmon production is farmed. At least in our supermarkets here in the UK, the cheapest fish available is now very often farmed salmon, certainly far cheaper than cod, halibut or mackerel! And in the fruit section are some apparent oddities such as persimmon, which you can get today but is hardly common, and muskmelon . . . which I had to Google, and turns out to be the variety of melons that encompasses cantaloupe and honeydew. Anyway, if you are a foodie like I am (and even if you are not), it is a very interesting read.

So where do the caloric values on food packaging, including on my packet of pork scratchings from The Bell pub in Bottisham,

come from? More than a century on, the vast majority of the caloric values are still largely based on Atwater's original factors.

THE HUMAN BODY AS A MACHINE

While Atwater's energy value factors made him a household name,
he was far from being a one-trick pony. He also performed critically important whole-body calorimetry experiments on humans
that were equally, if not more, important to our understanding of
human nutrition. Atwater visited Germany multiple times and
continued to follow Rubner's work even after he had moved from
Munich to Marburg. Rubner had, in 1884, built the world's first
'self-recording' whole-body calorimeter and used it on a dog to
demonstrate that the first law of thermodynamics did not only
hold true in machines, but that it was also true for animals. Atwater
knew immediately that he wanted to extend the work of Rubner
beyond dogs and into humans.

At the time, even after the work in dogs, people still did not
think that the first law of thermodynamics would hold true in
humans, because humans were, of course, 'unique' (the hubris
and self-importance of humans never fails to disappoint). In
1892, Atwater began a collaboration with his physicist colleague
Edward Bennett Rosa, designing and building what would become, in 1897, the Atwater–Rosa calorimeter.[13] Then between 1898
and 1900, Atwater conducted detailed experiments on four different healthy men (and, yes, they were all men), feeding them
different combinations of food, and getting them to do differing
amounts of exercise.[14] Like Rubner's previous experiments in dogs,
Atwater showed that whatever the men ate and breathed in was
used to keep the body running, producing, as a consequence, heat
and waste (solid, liquid or gaseous). If the men exercised harder, they used more energy; if they were sedentary, less energy was

used. Everything that went in = everything that came out, with no loss of energy. Thus, Atwater demonstrated that the first law of thermodynamics (that energy can be neither created nor destroyed), also functioned in humans. Well, to be accurate, Atwater actually only showed this in men, but future experiments following up his findings showed that, as expected, the same also held true in women and children.

The other odd thing that people thought at the time was that calories from different types of food were more or less effective for doing different types of work; so calories from carbohydrates were more useful for mechanical work, whereas calories from fat were more effective for heat, for example. As an ancillary to the primary finding that the conservation of energy held true in humans, Atwater showed that Rubner's 'isodynamic law' of calories (if you recall, this is the 'a calorie is a calorie' law) was also true in humans. From the moment a calorie was absorbed into the body, the law indicated it didn't matter where it came from, it would still enable exactly the same amount of work. Atwater also demonstrated, rather depressingly, that mental energy, i.e. thinking or calculating, did not use up calories. What about all the late-nighters I pulled while writing this book, fuelled by noodles, pork scratchings and gummy bears (sometimes all together in one sitting)? Are you saying it did nothing for my brain? That it all got converted to fat?! (Yes.)

Atwater even determined, somewhat controversially for the time, the energy value of alcohol to be 7 calories per gram, and demonstrated that alcohol calories were not inferior, and would fuel work exactly the same as calories from fat, carbs or protein.[15] This became an issue because the liquor trade made use of it in its advertising . . . I mean, why wouldn't they? The problem was that Atwater's employer and institution, Wesleyan University, was supported by the Methodist church. The church, at the time, was recommending total abstinence from alcohol (keeping in mind that this was just a scant couple of decades before Prohibition came into effect in America in 1920), with its members circulating pamphlets that described alcohol as nothing but poison. Just to be clear, alcohol is indeed a poison; most of us just happen to drink it in doses that are not harming us, or at least not killing us rapidly. As Paracelsus supposedly said, '*sola dosis facit venenum*', which is Latin for 'the dose makes the poison'. Atwater, ever the scientist, retorted that the Almighty would not wish moral teaching to be based on untruths. Hmmm . . . prescient words we might just wish to apply in the world we live in today.

Atwater's concern with metabolism went beyond physiology. He wanted to use his new techniques to determine improved dietary standards for the working class, standards that might prescribe a diet providing optimum food value at the lowest cost. Atwater believed that 'the cheapest food is that which furnishes the largest amount of nutriment at the least cost; and the best food is that which is both most healthful and cheapest'. His view was that as long as there was a balance between fat, carbs and protein, then the source of the food didn't matter. We will come back to assess this interesting view towards the end of this book.

Atwater's *Experiments on the Metabolism of Matter and Energy in the Human Body*, in which he reported all of these findings, was published in 1901,[16] and is still in print, I might add! I have, for one reason or another, been in the market for books about calories from the early twentieth century recently.

LULU HUNT PETERS AND CALORIE COUNTING

While Atwater had introduced the concept of calories as energy in food to scientists and policy makers in America, it wasn't until 1918 that a doctor from California brought it to the broader public consciousness. Lulu E. Hunt was born in 1873 to Thomas and Alice Hunt of Milford, Maine. After going to school in Maine, Lulu then moved to Los Angeles where she married Louis Peters in in 1899 and took the name Lulu Hunt Peters. She went to the University of California at Berkeley (my alma mater, Go Bears!), and graduated as a Doctor of Medicine in 1909. A remarkable achievement given the time, only sixty years on from when Elizabeth Blackwell became the first woman in either the UK or the US to receive a medical degree.

(Before I continue, you must forgive me for being vulgar enough to raise the issue of an individual's weight, particularly that of a woman. In this circumstance, I promise, it is relevant to our story.)

Peters always had an issue with her weight. She wrote:

'... *all my life I have had to fight the too, too solid. Why, I can remember when I was a child I was always being consoled by being told that I would outgrow it, and that when I matured I would have some shape. Never can I tell pathetically "when I was married I weighed only 118 (pounds), and look at me now". No, I was a delicate slip of 165 when I was taken.'*[17]

Peters actually reached her peak weight of 220 pounds (100 kilograms) soon after she graduated from medical school, and through some unspecified Damascene conversion, clearly felt the need to do something about it. So she began researching the latest publications on nutrition and metabolism in order to find a weight-loss solution for herself.

It was at this point that Atwater's work on calories and calorimetry showed up on her radar. Peters realised that if the first law of thermodynamics worked in humans, then the only way that she was going to lose weight was to eat less than she was burning, although this was hardly breaking news. The crucial difference was that Peters didn't just imagine what eating 'less' meant; rather, with her intellectual head on, she actually used the latest science to quantify and hence reduce the number of calories that she ate.

Thus, simply by rigorous calorie counting, Peters ended up losing an incredible 70 pounds (32 kilograms), and reaching what
she called her 'normal' weight of 150 pounds. As she was going
through this process, Peters converted all of the scientific and
technical information that she was gathering into lay-language,
and began a nationally syndicated newspaper column called 'Diet
and Health', which ran for many years in more than four hundred
papers. In 1918, Peters finally pulled all of the threads of her personal experience and her research together and *Diet and Health –
with key to the calories* was published. It was the very first popular
'diet book' and introduced 'the calorie' and the concept of calorie
counting to the general public.[18]

I say the 'general public', but in actuality the target audience of
Peters's book was (initially) the 'middle-class' American (almost
certainly white) woman *circa* 1918. Hold up, though. Was being
overweight even an issue in 1918? While obviously not anywhere
near the problem it is today, it was emerging as a middle-class
problem in the US. The industrial revolution had transformed the
face of America. The 'wild west' frontier, having reached California and the Pacific, was no more and cities were rapidly growing.
Even though the First World War was raging in Europe, and by
1917 the US had become deeply involved, it was still a distant war.
If anything, the war was somewhat of an economic boost to the
US. As a result, the excesses of modern living were beginning to
take their toll on the middle-class American woman, who, by and
large, still did not work.

An interesting aside was that in the early 1900s, corsets were
still in wide use by women in an effort to slim the body and make
it conform to whatever silhouette was fashionable at the time.
However, shortly after the US entered the First World War in
1917, American women were encouraged to stop buying corsets in
order to free up metal for war production. This single step was said
to have liberated some 28,000 tons of metal, enough to build two

battleships![19] That is a lot of difficulty breathing, body-slimming and silhouetting. As a result, the market for corsets bottomed out, and by the early 1920s, the corset had left the realm of common use and entered that of the costume drama. The problem was that without the mechanical aid to literally 'stay in shape', many women were now looking for natural ways to actually get into shape, which meant, sadly, to lose weight.

Thus, Peters's calorie-counting book, written in an accessible, conversational and actually very funny style, found fertile ground. She provided a rule for readers to find their ideal weight, some kind of prototype BMI calculation:

'Multiply number of inches over 5 feet in height by 5½; add 110. For example: Height 5 feet 7 inches without shoes. 7 × 5½ = 38½ + 110. Ideal weight 148½ pounds'.

Peters advised that in order to lose weight successfully, people needed to quantify the exact portion size of food they were eating.

'I have said that food, and food only, causes fat. That gives you the cue to what you must do to get rid of it . . . Hereafter you are going to eat calories of food. Instead of saying one slice of bread, or a piece of pie, you will say 100 calories of bread, 350 calories of pie'.

She then furnishes the reader with her rule of how to lose weight. The number of calories one needs when NOT trying to lose weight is, according to Peters, 15 to 20 calories (depending on how active one is) per pound of 'ideal weight'. So, if your ideal weight is 150 pounds, then an inactive person should be eating 15 × 150 = 2250 calories per day, whereas an active person should be eating 20 × 150 = 3000 calories per day. If the numbers seem surprisingly high, it's probably because everyone, including middle-class American women, was more active back in 1918 than most of us are today. Here is the critical part of the rule: in order to lose weight, you would then need to cut 500 to 1000 calories per day from your ideal caloric requirement. So an inactive person who was 5 feet 7 inches and should have an ideal weight of 148.5

pounds but currently weighed 220 pounds (Peters did not explicitly say so, but she was clearly using herself as an exemplar),
would need to be eating around 1200 calories a day in order to
lose weight. Peters, clearly familiar with the 'a calorie is a calorie'
law, paid less attention to what sorts of foods a person should eat,
save to maintain a 'balanced diet', even while calorie counting; in
other words, eat a little less of everything. Words to live by, even
more than a century on.

Crucially, Peters's advice was practical and actionable because
the book included estimates of hundreds of different food portions that would contain 100 calories, all pulled from Atwater's
many tables. Three ounces of roast beef, say, as long it was very
lean (she stresses), or a 1 ounce frankfurter sausage, or ½ ounce
of crispy bacon (damn you, bacon!), or 4 ounces of lobster, or one
hen's egg, or twenty large stalks of asparagus, or 3 ounces of boiled white potatoes, were all 100-calorie portions.

Along with presenting American women with a solution for
weight loss, it was interesting that, in the context of the First World
War, Peters sought to frame weight control as a form of patriotism.
Because rationing was a regular part of daily life during the war,
Peters suggested that her portion-control approach would make
dealing with rationing easier, and also help prevent food short-
ages. Thus, by counting calories, women could be patriotic and get
into shape at the same time! America needs you; just a little bit less
of you! It was a win–win!

Shortly after her book was published, Peters travelled to the
Balkans, where she served with the American Red Cross until
the end of the war and a couple of years into the recovery period.
When she returned, *Diet and Health – with key to the calories* had
become the first dieting book to become a bestseller, remaining
in the list of top-ten non-fiction books between 1922 and 1926,
and actually topping the list in 1924 and 1925.[20] All in all, it sold 2
million copies. In fact, it is still in print today, more than a hundred

years on. I found this out when I looked for it and ordered it online, adding to my collection of early twentieth-century calorie books and contributing, in the process, another half a penny (or whatever) to the Peters estate.

Lulu Hunt Peters successfully brought 'the calorie' into the public consciousness, where it has remained to this day. In linking those small units of energy to weight, either gain or loss, Peters had, in effect, 'weaponised' the concept of the calorie, and by doing so, sowed the seeds for the birth of an entire new industry.

PROBLEMS WITH THE ATWATER FACTORS

Atwater got many things right, but he also got a number of crucial things wrong when he was working out his factors. Just to be clear, I'm not 'dissing' Atwater and his achievements in any way. His work on calorimetry and his fuel value factors are, after all, more than a hundred and twenty years old! With all of the improvements in science and technology since then, it is amazing to me that his work on the calorie has stood as long as it has. Saying that, though, it is interesting that in *Principles of Nutrition and Nutritive Value of Food* Atwater did take a swipe at Rubner, saying that the Atwater factors 'are based upon the latest and most reliable research and take into account only the material which is digested and oxidised', as opposed to Rubner's estimates, which were 'based on less accurate data and not making allowance for the amounts of fats and carbohydrates which escape oxidation in the body'.[21] Meow.

Anyhow, while Atwater was correct in pointing out the flaws in Rubner's fuel-value estimates, the past 120 years have, in turn, revealed the flaws in Atwater's factors (and, just to be fair, Rubner's factors as well).

The first of these flaws was in the conversion factor used to estimate the total amount of protein from total nitrogen content. The nitrogen content of each of the amino acids (the protein building blocks) varies according to the molecular weight of the specific amino acid and the number of nitrogen atoms it contains, which can range from one to four, depending on the amino acid. Here's the thing, though, different sources of protein will have different compositions of amino acids. As I mentioned previously, Atwater based his conversion factor on the average amino acid composition of meat, which contains, on average 16 per cent nitrogen. When you divide 100 per cent by 16 per cent, you get a conversion factor of 6.25. The problem is that the nitrogen content of proteins actually varies from about 13 to 19 per cent. This would equate to nitrogen conversion factors ranging from 5.26 (100 per cent divided by 19 per cent) to 7.69 (100 per cent divided by 13 per cent), which would result in very different total protein amounts, and hence different calorie-counts. In response, in 1931 D.B. Jones suggested that universal use of the 6.25 factor be abandoned and replaced by food-specific factors.[22] These specific factors, now referred to as 'Jones factors', have been widely adopted. That being said, when taking the most widely eaten classes of food into consideration, then the range of Jones factors for major sources of protein in the diet is actually quite narrow. Meat-based protein retains its 6.25 conversion factor, cereal- and legume-based proteins have conversion factors in the range of 5.7 to 6.25, while dairy protein has a conversion factor of 6.38, for example.

The second major flaw was the calculation of carbohydrate content 'by difference', which, if you recall, meant that the other constituents in the food (protein, fat, water and ash) were first determined individually, added together and then subtracted from the total weight of the food. Whatever was left was assumed to be carbohydrates, which is largely correct. However, the problem is that this method groups ALL of the different carbohydrates together, from simple sugars to starch, to dietary fibre, to fibre we can't digest at all and poop out (for further fabulous fibre facts, please go to Chapter 7). So in 1970, a new factor of 3.75 calories per gram of simple sugar was added. And then in 1998, a further factor of 2 calories per gram of dietary fibre was recommended. These additions, when grouped together with Atwater's original three factors (four when you include alcohol) are known as the extensive general factor system.

Third, it is now clear that how, and in what proportions, proteins, fats and carbohydrates are mixed together within individual food items will influence the heats of combustion of the individual macronutrients. So, for example, because proteins differ in their amino-acid composition (as we have discussed), this can actually result in very different heats of combustion, with the heat of combustion of protein in rice (3.82 calories per gram), for instance, being around 20 per cent higher than that of protein in potatoes (2.78 calories per gram)! Equally, the digestibility and fibre content of food, such as wholewheat flour versus an extensively milled wheat flour, will have different available energy from equal amounts. Thus, the Atwater specific factor system – well, less of a system, and more of a series of tables – was created.[23] These were lists of various foods with substantial variability in the energy factors. So under this specific factor system, some examples of how widely the fuel values can differ between different foods are listed below:

- Eggs: 9.02 calories per gram of fat, 3.68 calories per gram of carbs and 4.36 calories per gram of protein;
- Meat/fish: 9.02 calories per gram of fat, 4.27 calories per gram of protein;
- Dairy: 8.79 calories per gram of fat, 3.87 calories per gram of carbs and 4.27 calories per gram of protein;
- White rice: 8.37 calories per gram of fat, 4.16 calories per gram of carbs and 3.82 calories per gram of protein;
- Potatoes: 8.37 calories per gram of fat, 4.03 calories per gram of carbs and 2.78 calories per gram of protein;

- Soybeans: 8.37 calories per gram of fat, 4.07 calories per gram of carbs and 3.47 calories per gram of protein.

If this is the kind of thing that rolls your socks down, then go to Appendix 1 to see a selected list of these specific factors.

So, taking a look at all of the different variations of fuel values, the specific factor system appears to be superior to the original Atwater general system – which took only protein, fat, total carbohydrate and alcohol into account, but, unlike the more extensive general factor system, does not take into account the differentiation between available carbohydrate and dietary fibre. In reality, though, because the specific factor system relies on lists, which are in practice cumbersome and yet quite limited in the types of foods that are included, Atwater's original 9–4–4 general factors are still overwhelmingly in use in the calorie information you read on your snack packet.

So going back to the equation:

A – The number of calories actually in the food ≠
B – The number of calories on the side of the pack ≠
C – The number of usable calories we finally get out of the food.

In this chapter, I have explained how we got from 'A', the total number of calories in a food as measured by bomb calorimetry, to 'B', the calorie-counts we see on most food packaging today. However, all three systems that we have discussed thus far (four if we include Rubner's estimations) do not take into account one critical factor: the loss of energy in heat as each of the different macronutrients are being chemically disassembled within the body in order to drive metabolism. In order to understand why and how and where this happens, and hence how we get to 'C', the final part of the equation, we first need to understand how we go about converting food into energy. And for that, we need to go to Chapter 3.

How do we turn food into energy?

'I like keeping my metabolism on its toes. Like what's it
gonna be today, complete starvation or 6,000 calories?'

Internet meme I thought was funny . . .

My wife, Jane, whom I've been married to for more than twenty
years, is an English rose. Now, at the risk of stereotyping the English people with big sweeping characterisations . . . Oh hell, I've
been here in Cambridge for more than twenty-five years, I am
almost English anyway, so let's jump in with some broad-stroke
stereotypes! (I will, however, not get myself into more trouble than
is necessary and leave the Scottish, Welsh and Northern Irish folk
out of this.) There are actually many 'non-English' characteristics
that Jane possesses: she has a sparkling, loud personality (not
unheard of for the English, the loud bit, but quite rare), she is
forthright in letting you know what she thinks (most definitely
not English) and she certainly has a full range of emotions (not
a stiff upper lip in sight). But, in many other ways, Jane is VERY
English: she calls her mother 'Mother' (not mom, mum, ma, mam,
mummy or a gazillion other contractions the rest of the world
seems to have managed to find); she needs her dinner plate heated
red hot, but her food not too hot (unlike the Chinese who tend
to have boiling hot food on cold dishes); she likes 'bread-sauce'
with her Christmas turkey dinner (this is mushy bread in warm
clove-flavoured salty milk . . . I'm not kidding, look it up); and
she loves gardening and/or walking in the rain (I mean she'd like

doing it not in the rain as well, but this is England and needs must).

However, what really makes her cast-iron, boilerplate-engraved, *bona fide* English is her love of a good cuppa tea. Now, all of us have had tea in some guise, at some point. Green tea, gunpowder black tea, iced tea with lemon, sun tea, spiced Indian chai tea, and even what you might have thought of as traditional English breakfast tea. But I guarantee you that unless you've had it here in England, you haven't actually had a cuppa; I've been here a long time now and am married to a local, so it has been (figuratively) beaten into me. Three components are essential: good quality black tea (when leaving the country, Jane actually travels with her own tea bags, because tea everywhere else seems to be a source of deep disappointment to her), fresh milk (not ultra-pasteurised milk as the French like, and certainly not cream or 'creamer' that the Americans prefer) and water on a rolling boil (it has to still be bubbling, and can't have been sitting around for any length of time after being boiled). The tea has to be made in a pot, and (this part wars have been fought over) you can either have the milk in the cup first before pouring in the tea, or you can pour the tea and then add the milk (Jane pours the milk first than the tea . . . don't @ me, I just make the tea and don't drink it; I'm a coffee man myself). As Jane always tells me, nothing cannot be fixed or solved with a good cuppa.

Anyway, one weekend morning, not so long ago, I was performing my domestic tea-making duties. So I filled the kettle with a litre of water, turned it on, and voila, about ninety seconds later, the essential water on a rolling boil. Now, having just spent the best part of two chapters contemplating 'heats of combustion', have you ever given any thought to the amount of energy it takes to actually get a kettle to boil? A calorie, as you now know, is the amount of energy it takes to raise 1 litre of water 1°C at sea level. Given that water boils at 100°C, then, think about it, it actually only takes 100 calories to boil a litre of water!! In fact, since the water came out of the tap, it was probably already at, I dunno, 15°C? Which means it only took 85 calories to get the litre of water from 15°C to boiling! If we consider how much 100 calories is in terms food, then that is probably only one medium-sized hen's egg, or less than half of a Mars bar. Given that most of us consume more than 2000 to 2500 calories a day, that is theoretically enough energy to heat up to 25 litres of water from freezing to boiling! Since we only have around 5 to 5.5 litres of blood flowing through us, how come we ourselves aren't literally boiling?

The answer is that living creatures, including humans, as demonstrated by Max Rubner and then Wilbur Atwater, conform to the first law of thermodynamics: the energy that we take in cannot be destroyed, but can be transferred or changed to another form. Thus, while there is clearly an awful lot of energy tied up in food, our body is able to take that raw energy, which if released all at once would indeed boil us, and gradually transform it into small units of transportable energy that can either be used immediately, or stored. This happens in two different steps. The first, which all of us know about, is the process of digestion. This gets food from your mouth, into your stomach, through to your intestines and then into the bloodstream. Many people think that is it; once food gets absorbed into the blood, we are then able to burn it like petrol or diesel or any other type of fuel. But it turns out to be a lot more complicated than that, because while digestion has indeed disassembled food into its component parts, which are dissolved in the blood and thus carried throughout the body, these component parts are just intermediaries. Crucially, depending on whether you are hungry or full, these intermediate components can either, respectively, be converted to usable energy or be stored in specific tissues for further use. This second step is the process called 'intermediary metabolism'.

THE DIGESTIVE SYSTEM

I happen to own a full-sized knitted replica of a human gut, because that is how I roll. It is, in effect, an anatomically correct (or as anatomically correct as something knitted is likely to be) uber-long woollen scarf, complete with organs made out of appropriately shaped cushions. Perhaps it might even take off as the latest 'it' thing for the autumn or winter collections from the big fashion houses; if we could only convince Lady Gaga to pair it with her 'meat dress' that she wore on the red carpet at the 2010 MTV Music Video Awards . . . Come on! What an ensemble that would be! Anyway, we can but dream. In the meantime, while awaiting the phone call from Lady Gaga and undoubted fame, I use the knitted gut as a prop for talks to audiences of all ages, calling it our food-to-poop tube. It always is incredibly popular, primarily because I say 'poop' multiple times (poop poop poop). It is unsurprising that kids find it funny, but the word, as it turns out, manages to tickle the puerile portion of all our brains, even when deeply buried within the recesses of the most staid and/or chronologically challenged of individuals (poop poop poop). And when you unfurl and stretch the knitted gut out, as I do whenever the space allows (and it needs a whole lot of space), it unfailingly elicits a collective intake of breath from the audience (myself included, and I've seen the thing a zillion times), because it is so very long, at around nine metres or thirty feet at full length.

The 'food-to-poop tube' is actually a surprisingly accurate description of our gastrointestinal tract or digestive system (Figure 1), which is, after all, a tube that takes food and extracts as many nutrients and as much water from it as possible before jettisoning the leftovers out the other end as poop. Starting at the food end, the digestive system begins with our mouth, which is connected via the oesophagus to our stomach; emerging from the stomach is the 'small' intestine, which at nearly six to seven metres long is by far the largest component of the system; this leads to the 'large' intestine (a misnomer at only one and a half metres long); ending with the rectum and finally the anus, the 'poop-chute'. In addition, there are a number of accessory organs that adorn this tube, salivary glands in the mouth, and the liver, gall-bladder and pancreas near the top of the small intestine. The amazing thing is that all nine metres of this is somehow origamied into our torso, without any kinks!

Figure 1

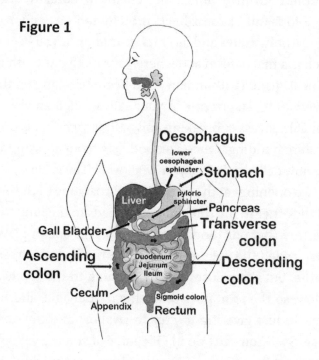

Digestion – from the mouth to the stomach

There are two types of digestion: mechanical digestion, which is literally the physical breaking down of food; and chemical digestion, which is, as the name suggests, a series of chemical reactions with different enzymes responsible for the breakdown of different food components. Mechanical and chemical digestion are not mutually exclusive of each other but work in concert. Let us imagine sitting down to a meal, and because I'm sat here writing this in Cambridge in the UK, let's go with something very typically English: Prime rib of beef roasted medium rare (mmmm . . . the king of cuts), Yorkshire pudding (done in a little beef fat, yum), roast potatoes (in goose fat, of course, double yum), beef jus, assorted steamed vegetables and horseradish sauce (oh gosh, I'm drooling . . . I know what I'm cooking this weekend).

Digestion, both mechanical and chemical, actually begins the moment a fork-full of roast beef (protein and fat) and Yorkshire pudding (carbohydrates and fat) hits your mouth. You begin chewing, which is a mechanical act, where your teeth cut (with incisors and canines), grind (with molars) and begin breaking up the food. At the same time, an enzyme in your saliva called amylase begins the chemical process of breaking down the starch that is present in the Yorkshire pudding. Once the food gets to an appropriate level of mush, now called a 'bolus', you swallow it. The issue is, there are actually two openings at the back of the throat, one to the oesophagus, and the other to the trachea, which leads to the lungs. How do we make sure that our food enters the correct opening? We have a little flap called the epiglottis, which normally stays open so we can breathe, but then closes up the opening to the trachea when we swallow, so the food goes down the oesophagus and heads to the stomach. Just give it a go, try to swallow and breathe at the same time. See? You can't do it! Of course, if you are yakking away or laughing while eating, or simply eating too quickly, the food sometimes goes down the wrong tube, and that is when you choke. This feels unpleasant when it is a small piece of food, normally leading to a coughing spasm to get the food out, but if the piece of food is large enough to block the trachea, preventing you from breathing, it can also clearly kill you, something that would most certainly ruin your day, and that you should probably avoid.

The oesophagus is really just a transit zone, moving the bolus of food from your mouth to your stomach, with the only digestion coming from the continued action of salivary amylase working on starch. Once the bolus gets to the bottom of the oesophagus, it encounters the 'lower oesophageal sphincter', which is a one-way system letting food and liquid enter the stomach, but not letting anything from the stomach come back out; or at least, that is what should happen. If the sphincter weakens, for a myriad of reasons, it can let acid from the stomach back into the oesophagus, that burns the delicate oesophageal wall, leading to the painful sensation we know of as 'heartburn'. If you didn't already know, 'heartburn' clearly has nothing whatsoever to do with the heart!

Once the sphincter lets the bolus past, it then enters the acidic cauldron that is the stomach. At a pH of 1.5, it really is quite a hostile environment (the lower the pH, the more acidic something is). By way of comparison, battery acid has a pH of 1.0. Here, the muscles of the tough, acid-resistant stomach walls mechanically churn the bolus in a process called peristalsis, not unlike a washing machine, mixing it with the digestive enzymes and gastric acids. One of the digestive enzymes that is secreted is a protein-digesting enzyme called pepsin. The gastric acids, which include hydrochloric acid, have two purposes: first, to kill the vast majority of unwelcome bacteria that enter the stomach; and second, to activate pepsin. Pepsin, like many enzymes, is produced in an inactive form, and is only made active when it is in the right place at the right time. You don't want pepsin to activate in, say, a cell, where it could begin to digest the proteins that are critical for the functioning of the cell. Pepsin requires the strong acidic conditions of the stomach to activate it, and in so doing begin the process of digesting protein found in the beef from its long complex chains of hundreds or thousands of amino acids to much shorter fragments. This process within the stomach continues for several hours, with the average human stomach comfortably holding about a litre of food, until the bolus of food becomes a partially digested liquid called chyme. Chyme is then slowly released by the pyloric sphincter, another one-way system, into the small intestine, for the next step of digestion.

Digestion – the small intestine

The small intestine can be anatomically divided into three sections: the uppermost part is the duodenum, which is the shortest structure, between twenty-five and forty centimetres long; the jejunum, which is the mid-section, and is between two and a half and three metres long; and the final section is the ileum, which is around three metres long. The inner wall of a typical healthy small intestine is covered in millions of 'villi', which are tiny finger-like projections about a half to one millimetre in size, depending on which section we're looking at; just imagine a shag-pile carpet that has been rolled up into a tube and you'd get a pretty good magnified idea of what it should look like. The villi act to increase the surface area through which the absorption of nutrients can occur. The surface area of a typical small intestine, when all stretched out, is thirty metres squared! In addition, each villus has a good blood supply and its surface is only one cell thick, which means that nutrients are absorbed easily and then rapidly carried away by the blood to other parts of the body.

The chyme is slowly released by the pyloric sphincter from the stomach into the duodenum. It is into this region of the small intestine that a number of accessory organs directly secrete enzymes and other substances, and where the vast majority of chemical digestion happens. The first thing that happens is the production, by the Brunner's glands within the duodenum wall, of a mucus-rich alkaline secretion containing bicarbonate, which together with a similarly alkali solution secreted from the pancreas, neutralises the highly acidic chyme that has just emerged from the stomach. This is crucial, first to prevent the stomach acid from otherwise damaging the delicate villi of the small intestine, and second because all of the other enzymes and substances require a neutral pH to function appropriately. Bile, which is made by the liver and stored in the gall bladder, is then released into the duodenum to emulsify any fat in the beef and any that was used to cook the Yorkshire pudding. Fat, as you know, can't dissolve in water, and so bile acts pretty much like soap, breaking the large globs of fat into microscopic globules called micelles. This process greatly increases the surface area to volume ratio of the globules, hence allowing enzymes more efficient access to digest the fat. A whole suite of digestive enzymes are then released by the pancreas; pancreatic lipases begin the breakdown of the micelles of fat; pancreatic amylases take over from the salivary amylase (which has long since been destroyed by the stomach acids) to continue digesting carbohydrates; and chymotrypsin and trypsin take over from pepsin (which was deactivated once the acidic chyme was neutralised by the bicarbonate) in digesting the chains of protein into individual amino acids. It's a busy ol' place, the duodenum!

The increasingly digested food then enters the jejunum, which is where the vast majority of nutrient absorption occurs. It is here that the villi are longest; in fact, the cells that line these villi possess even larger numbers of microvilli (so there are villi upon villi . . . it all sounds like a Dr Seuss tale) to maximise the surface area for absorption. At this point, most of the beef and Yorkshire pudding have been digested into their constituent parts. Complex carbohydrates such as starches have been broken down to simple sugars such as glucose, and these will now be absorbed into the bloodstream. It is the same situation for proteins, which have now been digested into individual amino acids, and are subsequently transported across the wall of the intestine and into the blood.

Fat, however, is a more complicated beast, largely because it can't, unlike sugars and amino acids, be dissolved in water, which primarily forms what is in the gut and, of course, is what blood is made of. A different strategy is required, therefore, to move fat about the body. The fat that we eat and, as you will see later, store, is primarily in the form of 'triglycerides'; this is a backbone of a simple molecule called 'glycerol', on which three fatty acids are attached, hence the name triglyceride. The enzymes that digest fat are called lipases. Where does the name 'lipase' come from? You would have heard the term 'lipids' being used, sometimes interchangeably with 'fat'. Lipids are actually a broad group of molecules (wax, steroids and cholesterol, for instance, are all lipids), some playing a key role in the structural integrity of the cell wall, and that includes fat. So the 'lip' in lipase comes from lipid. As for the suffix 'ase', this will always indicate that the role of a particular enzyme is to break molecules down. Amylase, for example, comes from the Latin word *amylum* for starch, hence amylases are enzymes that break down starch. In the same way, proteases, such as pepsin and trypsin, are enzymes that break down protein, and lipases, well, they break down lipids, including fat.

As the micelles of fat navigate toward the villi on the intestinal wall, they are met by a lipase secreted from the pancreas. The lipase sits at the surface of the micelle, breaking each triglyceride down into three molecules of free fatty acids and either mono- or diglycerides, which are then moved into the cells that form the villi on the gut wall. Within these gut villi cells, the free fatty acids and glycerides are then reassembled into triglycerides, packaged into structures called chylomicrons, and moved into the blood stream to be transported elsewhere. 'What a convoluted procedure!' I know some of you are thinking, but this is what it takes to move fat within a largely water-based medium. We will find out the fate of the chylomicrons and their cargo of triglycerides later in the chapter.

Not all nutrients are able to be absorbed by everybody in the same way, though. An example of this is lactose, the primary sugar found in dairy products. Lactose is a disaccharide, meaning it is formed of two monosaccharides, in this case glucose and galactose. Sucrose, the powdered white stuff we actually know as sugar, is another example of a disaccharide, made of one molecule each of fructose and glucose. Most sucrose is split into fructose and glucose by the acid in our stomach, with the rest being digested by the enzyme sucrase that resides in the villi of the duodenum, and all humans deal with sucrose with similar effectiveness. Digestion of lactose, however, occurs entirely in the small intestine, which produces an enzyme called lactase-phlorizin-hydrolase, or simply 'lactase', that breaks down lactose into glucose and galactose before it is absorbed into the bloodstream. Most of the world, however, myself included, can't drink and eat dairy products, or more specifically can't digest lactose, as adults. This so-called 'lactose intolerance' is actually somewhat of a misnomer. All human infants, all very young mammals actually, drink milk as the major energy source and are therefore lactose tolerant in early life; this is what defines us as mammals, after all. Most mammals, including most humans, then become increasingly lactose intolerant in the transition to adulthood. This is caused when another protein comes along and binds to a segment of DNA next to the *Lactase* gene, and in doing so, turns the gene off, stopping the production of lactase. This is why I, for example, am unable to drink milk. However, around 7500 years ago, when the first dairy herds were domesticated in Europe, a mutation emerged in humans that prevented the protein that turned off the *Lactase* gene from binding to the adjacent segment of DNA; thus lactase is never turned off.[1] Being able to drink milk and eat dairy products as a source of calories would have been a huge selective advantage in a time when there would not have been enough food, so the mutation became fixed in Northern Europeans. Today, 85 per cent of people of Northern European extraction can drink milk as adults, and all have this exact same mutation that came into Europe some 7500 years ago. In the rest of the world, such as in China where my ancestors came from, because dairying was not a big thing, the selection pressure was not there for us to adapt to be able to drink milk in adulthood. Thus there are differing abilities in our digestive systems to be able to deal with lactose, with some of us having to run to the loo after eating cheese a little more quickly than others.

The final stage for what is left of our meal is to enter the last section of the small intestine. The ileum is about three metres long, and contains villi similar to the jejunum, where it absorbs mainly vitamin B12 and bile acids, as well as any other remaining nutrients that were not absorbed by the jejunum. Layers of circular and longitudinal smooth muscle produce waves of muscle contractions called peristalsis. While in the stomach this causes a washing-machine-type movement, in the ileum it pushes the remnants of our digested meal in one direction, towards the large intestine.

Digestion – the large intestine

The large intestine is about one and a half metres in length and subdivided into six sections. The ileum of the small intestine empties into the 'cecum', a small antechamber of sorts, which includes the appendix. It then heads almost immediately up into the 'ascending colon', turns right at the liver into the 'transverse colon', heads down again just past the spleen into the 'descending colon', takes a bit of a wiggle through the 'sigmoid colon', before entering the 'rectum', and getting to the exit at the anus. By the time the chyme emerges into the cecum, most nutrients and 90 per cent of the water have been absorbed. With all of the chemical digestion completed in the small intestine, the large intestine produces no digestive enzymes. At this point what is left are the indigestible remnants of the meal including, crucially, dietary fibre, which is primarily indigestible carbohydrate in either soluble or insoluble form. We will come back to the importance of this seemingly waste product in Chapter 6. As peristalsis moves the chyme through the large intestine, it is mixed with mucus and gut bacteria and becomes faeces. This material is initially liquid as it moves up the ascending colon, but as it travels through the rest of the colon, all of the excess water is absorbed, causing the stools to gradually solidify as they move along into the descending colon. And voila, we have wondrous, fabulous poop.

Of course, as all of us know, some poop is less *ahem* solid than others. This can happen for a myriad of different reasons, including illness or food poisoning or even a disagreeable meeting between a new type of food and your resident gut bacteria. On occasion, I go to Mexico to teach at the Cuernavaca campus of the Universidad Nacional Autónoma de Mexico (UNAM). I am a huge fan of spicy food and love chillis, so the first time I was there, I was very excited to try out some of the different varieties of Mexican chillis. Whoooo, boy . . . can I tell you, did my gastrointestinal tract have an opinion about that! I have, like most people, suffered from food poisoning before, and this was not that type of explosive response. It was just that the introduction of a different type of chilli, and I'm normally fine with all manner of chillis, clearly re-sulted in the denizens of my gut deciding to go on strike. Another reason for fluctuating poop consistency may be intolerance to a particular nutrient, such as lactose, that we discussed above. If a large amount of undigested lactose, due to a lack of lactase activity ten to fifteen feet up north in the jejunum, makes it into the colon, two things happen to cause trouble. First, there is not normally a whole lot of sugar in faecal matter, but when there is, less water is absorbed by the gut, therefore causing the faeces to be less solid or not solid at all; second, the bacteria that reside in the colon begin to ferment the lactose, thus producing gas. This results in the characteristic gastrointestinal symptoms of lactose intolerance, which include abdominal bloating (a feeling of uncomfortable

fullness in the abdomen), often leading to abdominal pain, diar-
rhoea, gas and sometimes even nausea. These unpleasant effects
typically occur in lactose-intolerant individuals (like *moi*), between thirty minutes to two hours after consuming milk or milk
products. Symptoms can range from mild to severe depending
on the amount of lactose that has been consumed and also the
amount a person can tolerate. Which is why I, mostly not a sucker
for punishment, drink black americanos and not cappuccinos.

ATP – THE ENERGY CURRENCY OF LIFE

However, while glucose, fatty acids and amino acids are indeed
the individual deconstructed components of the food that we eat,
they are not, in and of themselves, actually units of energy. They
are easily transportable intermediaries. Once they are moved to
whatever tissue or organ they are destined for, they are then metabolised into units of usable energy. The energy 'currency' for
ALL life on earth is adenosine triphosphate, or ATP.

The perennial issue with the production of energy, is that if
not used, then either it is wasted or there needs to be an effective
and easily accessible storage solution. Let's take a country's electricity supply as an example. Electricity usage is not stable over a
twenty-four-hour period; there is higher demand during the day
when most people are awake, and naturally far lower use overnight. Even during the day there will be peaks and troughs in demand, with a spike in the morning when everyone boils water for
their hot caffeinated beverage, and in the evening when dinner is
being prepared. There are also less regular but equally predictable
spikes, such as if a country's football or rugby or ice-hockey team
is playing in an important international fixture, with a significant
proportion of the population tuned in to watch on television.
When half-time comes, everyone gets up, perhaps to use the loo,

turning on the light in the bathroom in the process, or running to the kitchen to grab a hot drink (requiring use of the kettle) or a cold beer (requiring the opening of a fridge), resulting in a very large spike in energy usage, but over a very short space of time. How does an electricity grid manage? Well, power stations can obviously increase or decrease energy production as necessary, but in the evenings, there will always be an excess of electricity being generated. There is also the rapidly increasing production of renewable energy from windfarms or tidal (and other marine) power generators that don't follow day/night cycles to consider. What happens to energy that is not used immediately? Well, the world's largest form of storage for excess electricity, however it is generated, is 'pumped hydroelectric energy storage'. This is when excess electricity, typically at night (but any time demand is low), is used to pump water from a lower reservoir to an upper reservoir based up on a hillside, where it is stored as 'potential energy'. Then during a World Cup final football match between England and Germany, say (we can but dream), when the half-time put-the-kettle-on-for-a-cuppa surge is approaching, an engineer simply turns on the tap, and the water flows down from the upper to the lower reservoir through hydroelectric turbines, thereby generating kinetic energy in the form of electricity. This electricity supply is temporary, but enough to cope with the half-time increase in demand. The water is then pumped back up the hill when there is spare capacity, awaiting the next anticipated surge. It is, in effect, an enormous, mountain-sized rechargeable battery.

Consider ATP a molecular-sized rechargeable battery. ATP (see Figure 2) is formed of two parts: the adenosine section (the part with three rings and nitrogen), and the 'triphosphate' or 'three phosphate' section. Instead of storing potential energy at the top of a hill, ATP stores energy within its chemical bonds, specifically within the triphosphate part. A phosphate is a molecule made of one phosphorous atom and four oxygen atoms, and the key thing

Figure 2

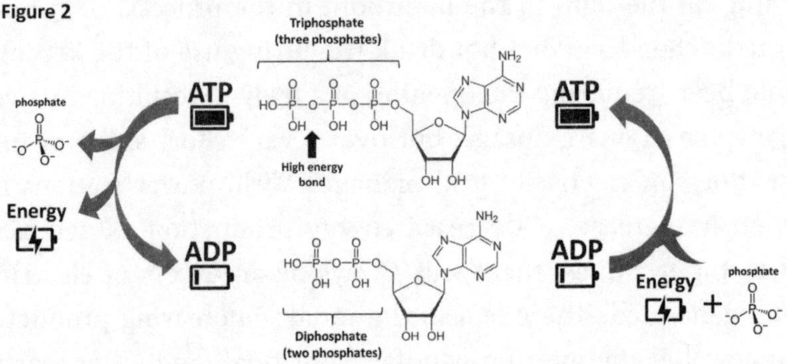

is it takes a lot of energy to drive the chemical reaction joining one phosphate molecule to another. But, through the first law of thermodynamics, we now know that energy doesn't just disappear but is transformed, and in this situation the energy is transferred into the bond holding the two phosphate groups together. So, when the reaction is reversed, and the two phosphate groups are separated, that energy is then subsequently released. Ultimately, the entire purpose of metabolising glucose, fatty acids and amino acids (we will look at how this happens later) is to generate the required energy to add a phosphate molecule onto Adenosine **di**phosphate (two phosphates) or ADP, converting it to Adenosine **tri**phosphate (three phosphates) or ATP. This stores the potential energy within the bond, keeping the second and third phosphate in ATP together. So if we stick with the analogy of a battery, then ADP could be considered 'empty' and needing recharging, while ATP would be a fully charged battery. These fully charged molecular batteries are present throughout every one of the thirty-seven trillion cells that make up our body. Then, whenever required, ATP loses its third phosphate and is converted back to ADP, a process that releases a small usable burst of energy. ADP is then free again to receive energy from the metabolism of glucose, fatty acids and amino acids to 'recharge' back to ATP, and the process repeats over and over.

This recycling of ATP is the universal energy currency for ALL life on Earth (we'll have to see what happens in alien life-forms when we bump into them). In our own bodies, ATP powers all our muscles, our heart (which is a special type of muscle, because it can't get tired and it never stops . . . until it does, of course), every single neuron in our brain, our immune system, our food to poop tube, our liver, our pancreas, our kidneys, our lungs, everything. ATP floats throughout each cell, like oxygen in the air, and is used every second of every day. In fact, on an average day, an average human being will use up to 50 to 75kg of ATP, with each ATP recycled (ATP to ADP and back to ATP again) 500 to 750 times. That is roughly our bodyweight, or around $6 \times 10^{25} - 9 \times 10^{25}$ (a '6' or '9' followed by twenty-five zeroes) molecules of ATP every single day in order to keep everything in our body ship-shape and ticking along.

METABOLISM, THE PRODUCTION OF ATP

When glucose, fatty acids and amino acids enter the bloodstream, they undergo one of two fates. Depending on our body's nutritional state, they are either metabolised to produce ATP, or they are stored for future use.

OK, so starting with metabolism, how do we get from the intermediate nutrients of glucose, fatty acids and amino acids to the production of ATP? Well, all life on Earth is carbon-based. Yes, there are numerous other elements that are crucial, such as oxygen (O), hydrogen (H), nitrogen (N), and phosphorus (P), but nearly every single molecule in ALL life, has a carbon backbone. You might look at the structure of ATP/ADP and say, hang on, I only see O, H, N and P? But, where each straight line meets and there isn't an O, H, N or P, then it is actually a carbon (C). There are so many carbons in organic-based molecules, including of course glucose, fatty acids and amino acids, that scientists don't even bother writing in the 'C's. Antoine Lavoisier showed all those years ago that burning carbon in the form of diamond or charcoal, in the presence of oxygen, released large amounts of energy in the form of heat and produced carbon dioxide as a waste product. He then realised, through his calorimetry studies, that the metabolism of nutrients, while a gentler and far less violent process, was essentially the same thing. Carbon-based glucose, fatty acids and amino acids are similarly 'burnt' in the presence of oxygen (which we breathe in), producing carbon dioxide (which we breathe out), but instead of releasing the energy all in one fell swoop as heat (which would then literally boil our blood), the energy is parcelled up into trillions upon trillions of ATP, allowing it to be directed and deployed in a controlled fashion.

I have summarised the process, called intermediary metabolism, as best as I can, in Figure 3. I appreciate it might look horrendously complex . . . and everyone who has studied biochemistry at any level would have had to at some point memorise some or all of the pathways (and, for the sake of simplicity, I've only listed a small fraction of the pathways). However, unless you are interested in the intricacies of the individual reactions from an academic perspective, it becomes unnecessarily complicated to go into the minutiae. Just for full disclosure, I studied biochemistry as an undergrad at UC Berkeley, and so I did, at some point, have the pathways memorised to make sure I passed my exams; which I did, otherwise I wouldn't be here. But I swear, the moment I stepped out of the exam hall, all the information evaporated, almost instantly, from my brain. What a waste of perfectly good ATP. Today, even if you put a gun to my head, I would not be able to draw out any of the pathways for you from memory! That being said, while the specific metabolites and enzymes are esoteric to many and difficult to memorise (it certainly was for me), the actual concept can be understood without having to go into the minutiae. Bear with me as I take you briefly (relatively speaking) through the basic principles of intermediary metabolism, highlighting some of the key components as we go along.

Figure 3

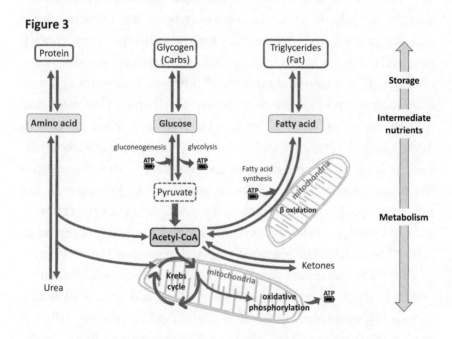

Glucose, fatty acids and amino acids all take different journeys to begin with, however, they eventually meet at a common mid-point, the generation of a molecule called **acetyl-CoA**, and from there on share a universal pathway that results in the production of ATP. You can consider acetyl-CoA to be the equivalent of coal to be shovelled into the furnace of a power station, and the power stations in each of our cells are the mitochondria. This seems as good a place as any to start our tour around intermediary metabolism.

MITOCHONDRIA, OUR CELLULAR POWER STATIONS

Every cell in our body, with the exception of our red blood cells, contain mitochondria. Cells don't only have one mitochondrion (the singular); rather, depending on the cell type, they contain hundreds or even thousands of mitochondria (the plural). Mitochondria play a role in a number of different important cell processes, including cell division (where a cell splits into two), cell differentiation (what a cell ends up becoming – a muscle cell? A kidney cell? A neuron?) and cell death (not dying because of disease, but 'programmed' death of an older cell, so that the components can be recycled). Its most important role, however, its day job, so to speak, is to generate energy. A significant proportion of the cell's energy is released as heat, playing a key role in keeping us warm, but mostly, the energy is released in the form of ATP.

Three key processes occur within the mitochondria when it comes to the production of energy. The first is the route by which fatty acids are broken down into acetyl-CoA, a process called 'β oxidation'; this we will look at later. The second and third are the Krebs cycle and oxidative phosphorylation respectively; these are two closely linked pathways that glucose, fatty acid and amino-acid metabolism eventually converge on, and are responsible for the conversion of acetyl-CoA into ATP. Ultimately, it is this processing of acetyl-CoA by the Krebs cycle and oxidative phosphorylation that powers most organs in the human body.

THE KREBS CYCLE

The Krebs cycle and oxidative phosphorylation might be paired, but each plays a very distinct role (Figure 4). The Krebs cycle, also known as the citric-acid cycle, is so called because it was discovered by Sir Hans Adolf Krebs in 1937, for which he received the Nobel Prize in Medicine in 1953.[2] Why should you care about the Krebs cycle? Well, the energy that is available from the breakdown of organic molecules is actually stored in the bonds that hold the carbon backbone of a cell together. So when you light charcoal for a BBQ, or burn petrol or diesel in an internal combustion engine to power your vehicle, or use gas for your boiler to heat your house and water, all of which are organic carbon-based fuels, the release of energy in the form of heat comes from the breaking of carbon bonds, with the liberated carbon combining with oxygen to form carbon dioxide. The actual process of burning, however, is clearly too uncontrolled and releases too much heat all at once to occur safely in living organisms. Enter the Krebs cycle, which is essentially a more gentle and controlled way of breaking carbon bonds in the food that we eat and hence liberating the locked-up potential energy for use within the oxidative phosphorylation pathway. But I am getting ahead of myself.

The Krebs cycle (Figure 4) begins (as far as any cycle has a beginning or an end) when **acetyl-CoA** is fed in, and the acetyl group, a two-carbon molecule, reacts with the four-carbon **oxaloacetate**, to form a six-carbon molecule, citrate, which is why Krebs called it the 'citric-acid cycle' (others later named it after Krebs . . . he wasn't quite that narcissistic). Then follow a further nine steps, whereby in the presence of oxygen, two carbons are sequentially removed from citrate and released as two molecules of carbon dioxide or CO_2, and are eventually converted back to oxaloacetate when another molecule of acetyl-CoA is fed in, and the cycle begins again. Carbon dioxide, as mentioned previously, is not the purpose of the cycle, it is a by-product, like exhaust from a vehicle. The purpose of the Krebs cycle is to produce electrons, which are, together with oxygen, then used to power oxidative phosphorylation and generate ATP (see next page).

Every atom has a nucleus of protons and neutrons, with protons having a positive electric charge (+ve) and neutrons, as its name suggests, having a neutral charge. This nucleus is then orbited by a corresponding number of electrons, which are negatively charged (–ve). Because the number of electrons in an atom typically balances out the number of protons, any given atom tends to have a neutral charge. An atom, however, can gain or lose an electron or two, without changing too much of its fundamental characteristics, except its charge. So hydrogen, for instance, is composed of one proton and one electron (it is the only atom without a neutron), so the +ve charge of the proton balances the –ve charge of the electron. If hydrogen loses its electron, then it becomes a proton or H^+, which has a +ve charge. This is important because if a cell can generate an electrical gradient by moving protons and electrons about, well, it can then generate energy.

Electrons, however, don't just ping about freely (they would just cling to everything, and nothing orderly would happen), but require carriers. The two electron carriers used by the Krebs cycle are NAD^+/NADH and $FADH/FADH_2$. When NAD^+ and FADH react with water, they are converted to NADH and $FADH_2$ respectively, and are now each carrying a package of two electrons that can be donated elsewhere. Each acetyl-CoA, by going through the Krebs cycle, will generate three molecules of NADH and one of $FADH_2$. NADH and $FADH_2$ then carry their cargo of electrons over to the Oxidative Phosphorylation pathway.

OXIDATIVE PHOSPHORYLATION AND THE GENERATION OF ATP

The mitochondria have an outer membrane that is relatively smooth, an intermembrane space, and an inner membrane that is definitely not smooth, more like crinkled-up Christmas wrapping paper, all wrapped around an internal chamber at the centre called the matrix. It is here, in the mitochondrial matrix, that the Krebs cycle takes place. While the role of the Krebs cycle is to break apart carbon bonds to release energy, it is the responsibility of 'oxidative phosphorylation' to use that energy to generate ATP. The crinkled-up bits of the inner mitochondrial membrane are called cristae, and it is on this membrane, through five large protein complexes, that 'oxidative phosphorylation' occurs (Figure 4). The term 'oxidative' means driven by oxygen, 'phosphorylation' means to add a phosphate group, and this oxygen-driven process just happens to add a phosphate group to ADP, converting it to ATP.

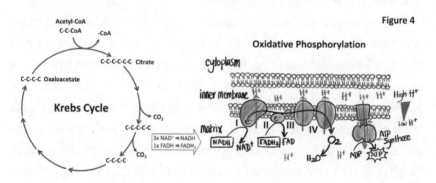

Figure 4

The first four of the large protein complexes that take part in oxidative phosphorylation are called, in a disappointing failure of imagination, complex I, II, III and IV. NADH and $FADH_2$ drop off their electrons at complexes I and II, and are oxidised by oxygen (O_2) back to NAD^+ and FADH, producing water in the process. The electrons travel from complex I through to IV, a little like electricity, but instead of passing through a wire, they are carried along by molecular shuttles between complexes; this is known as the 'electron transport chain'. Complexes I to IV, together with the electron transport chain, form the mitochondrial respiratory chain. The oxygen-driven electron transport chain powers complexes I, III and IV to pump protons (H^+) from the matrix, across the inner mitochondrial membrane through to the intermembrane space. This is equivalent to the 'pumped hydroelectric energy storage' analogy that I used previously, where water is pumped using electricity from a lower reservoir to a reservoir up in the hill, and stored as potential energy. When water is released back down the hill, its potential energy is converted into electrical energy as it flows through hydroelectric turbines. In the mitochondria, potential energy is clearly not water stored at a height and subject to the perils of gravity; rather its potential energy is stored as an electrical gradient, generated by a large positive charge from the accumulation of all those protons in the intermembrane region and a negative charge in the matrix.

This is where the fifth complex in oxidative phosphorylation, ATP synthase (hallelujah, it's not called complex V!), enters our story. A 'synthase' is an enzyme that drives a reaction to produce a substance; hence ATP synthase is the enzyme that produces ATP. ATP synthase looks and acts remarkably like a turbine. It has a fat stem and tulip-shaped head that actually spins, and unlike complexes I to IV it points in the opposite direction, into the matrix. When enough of a positive electrical gradient is reached, protons flow through ATP synthase from the intermembrane region into the matrix. In doing so, it powers the spinning head of the synthase, acting much like a hydroelectric turbine, which adds a phosphate group to each ADP, converting it to ATP. Each complete spin of the head of ATP synthase produces three ATP. All that oxygen we are breathing in? It is primarily to power respiration and the production of ATP. That is why the mitochondria, which 'burn' carbon in the presence of oxygen, are considered, quite literally, our cellular power stations. **The Krebs cycle and oxidative phosphorylation, ultimately, are the critical processes that convert the food we eat into calories.** Peter Mitchell from the University of Cambridge described how the respiratory chain worked to generate an electrical gradient (and the highly related process that happens in photosynthesis) and hence to produce ATP, in the early 1960s, receiving the Nobel Prize in Chemistry for the discovery in 1978.[3] In the late 1970s Paul Boyer from Los Angeles worked out specifically how ATP synthase worked, and John Walker, from Cambridge, figured out what its structure actually looked like, including the remarkable spinning head 'turbine' that spits out ATP, and both received the Nobel Prize in Chemistry in 1997.[4] All in all, a total of three Nobel prizes for the amazing discoveries of the Krebs cycle and oxidative phosphorylation.

The inner membrane of a single mitochondrion can contain over 10,000 sets of these respiratory chains and ATP synthase; a cell can contain many hundreds, even thousands of mitochondria; and there are around 37 trillion cells in the human body. That is how we manage to generate and go through our own bodyweight in ATP every single day!

CARBOHYDRATE METABOLISM

Each of the intermediate nutrients finds their way to becoming acetyl-CoA in very different ways, resulting in the production of different amounts of ATP. There are two ways of making your way through the next few sections. I will give you the bottom line first – how many ATP are produced per molecule of sugar or fat, say. That is sufficient info for most. However, I then follow the bottom line with a more detailed explanation . . . the 'how and why', for those of you that care!

Arguably the most straightforward is the metabolism of carbohydrates. Carbohydrates encompass a wide array of compounds, from fibre (which is largely undigested so flies right through the system and out the other side), to starch, to a large variety of sugars. The term 'sugar' encompasses many different compounds; glucose, fructose, lactose, galactose, sucrose . . . most compounds ending in '-ose', essentially. The powdered and granulated form that is most commonly used, found in food and available in shops, is sucrose, a disaccharide made from one molecule of each mono-saccharide glucose and fructose joined together. Lactose is also a disaccharide, made from glucose and galactose. Starch, in contrast, is a polysaccharide, made up of long chains of glucose molecules. Carbohydrates need to be digested down to monosaccharides in order to be absorbed. Since most of the carbohydrates that we consume are in the form of starch, the vast majority of carbohy-drates that come across the gut wall and into the bloodstream are glucose.

So the bottom line is that each molecule of glucose produc-es a total of thirty ATP when metabolised in the presence of oxygen.

Once glucose gets taken up by a cell, it is either stored (but only by certain types of cells) or it is metabolised (which can happen in all cells). The first part of glucose metabolism is a process called glycolysis (from 'glycose', an older term for glucose, and 'lysis' for degradation), in which a molecule of glucose is broken down into two molecules of **pyruvate** (Figure 3). Our energy currency is ATP, so every single thing that we do, or that happens within our bodies, can be considered to either 'cost' or 'earn' ATP. Through that prism, glycolysis uses up two ATP-worth of energy to break down every molecule of glucose, but generates four ATP in return, giving a net earning of two ATP; at the same time it also trans-fers electrons to two NAD^+, thus converting it into two NADH (which as we see above, powers oxidative phosphorylation to generate ATP). What is critical is that glycolysis is an 'anaerobic' process, meaning it can take place in the absence of oxygen. This is very useful for when there is little or no oxygen about (not a long-term situation clearly, but it does happen, as I explain later). The problem is that without oxygen, only two ATP are released per glucose molecule, because NADH can only generate ATP through 'oxidative' phosphorylation if oxygen is present. If NADH is not used, it then does not recycle back to NAD^+ to receive more electrons, and glycolysis would eventually stop. So what happens instead is that pyruvate is converted to lactate, and in doing so converts NADH back to NAD^+ to continue supplying glycolysis. When you are doing high-intensity physical activity, such as lifting anything heavy, or climbing multiple flights of stairs, or sprinting a short distance, you often can't get oxygen to the muscles fast enough, so this is called anaerobic activity. The ATP used to power that anaerobic physical activity will come initially from glycolysis, which produces lactate. Lactate spontaneously converts to lactic acid, which is what causes that burning sensation you feel in your muscles. Glycolysis is fine for high-intensity but short-duration activity. However, for any activity lasting longer than one minute, glycolysis simply does not produce enough energy fast enough. On top of that, lactic acid takes time to clear from the muscles, and if too much builds up, it simply becomes too painful for the muscles to function effectively. That is when the magic ingredient of oxygen has to be introduced, converting anaerobic activity to an aerobic activity.

In the presence of oxygen, each molecule of pyruvate is then converted to acetyl-CoA, which is transported to the mitochondria and enters the Krebs cycle, producing NADH and $FADH_2$ to feed oxidative phosphorylation. In addition, because no more lactate is being formed (because all the pyruvate is being used), you can also add the NADH made during glycolysis to the mix. So how much energy emerges from this aerobic process? Well, each NADH that is fed into oxidative phosphorylation generates two and a half ATP and each $FADH_2$ generates one and a half ATP. So if you tot everything up, the addition of oxygen to the mix produces an additional twenty-eight ATP!

In summary, there are two steps to how our body extracts energy from glucose. The first step, glycolysis, in which glucose is converted to pyruvate, doesn't use oxygen and produces a net of two ATP. It is very quick to activate and is used for short bursts of activity. The second step introduces oxygen, igniting the whole process, converting pyruvate to acetyl-CoA, which then enters the Krebs cycle and oxidative phosphorylation, and produces an additional twenty-eight ATP. Add that to the two ATP produced during glycolysis, then each molecule of glucose produces a total of thirty ATP with the involvement of oxygen; fifteen times more than simply relying on glycolysis.

MAKING GLUCOSE

In some situations, largely within the liver (and also the kidneys), pyruvate can be, at the cost of four ATP and two NADH, converted back to glucose. This process is known as gluconeogenesis (meaning new glucose formation) and the pathway is essentially the reverse of glycolysis. Why might your body need this facility? Well, the liver plays a number of key roles within the body. Most famously, it is the body's detox organ: with one to two litres of blood flowing through it every minute, the liver clears the blood of any toxins. However, many of you might not be aware that the liver's most important role is actually to make sure that your blood glucose levels do not drop too low. Blood glucose levels in someone without diabetes are maintained between four and seven millimolar. Just a quick primer, 1 'mole' is 6.02×10^{23} ('6' followed by twenty-three zeros) molecules of any substance, and 1 'molar' is 1 mole of a given substance dissolved in 1 litre of water; a millimolar would therefore be a thousandth of that. If blood glucose goes too high, then insulin gets secreted by the pancreas, and glucose gets taken up primarily by fat and the muscles. If the blood glucose goes too low, such as during periods of fasting, starvation, or intense exercise, and there is a danger of hypoglycaemia (low blood glucose), then the liver begins the process of gluconeogenesis to nudge glucose levels back into the safe zone.

Where does the starting material come from for the liver to make glucose? Some of it comes from the breakdown of certain amino acids, particularly in starvation situations (we look at this later), but quite a bit of it actually comes from lactate. Lactate is made in the muscles from pyruvate, when there are low local levels of oxygen. But eventually oxygen gets to the muscles, and lactate is then transported by the bloodstream to the liver, where it is converted back to pyruvate. The pyruvate is converted back to glucose by gluconeogenesis, and is then sent back to the muscles to be used to fuel glycolysis. This is known as the Cori cycle.

So pyruvate, depending on the nutritional status of the body, can either be metabolised completely to produce ATP, or it can be converted back to glucose. It is an important decision point, because the moment pyruvate becomes acetyl-CoA, it can no longer be converted back to glucose. This is important, particularly for the liver, because of its critical job of maintaining blood glucose levels in times of fasting or starvation, which it can only do when there is enough pyruvate about.

BREAKING DOWN FAT

Then we have fat, which is our long-term energy store. Fat is stored as triglycerides, which are three fatty-acid chains stuck on a glycerol backbone. Because fat is not soluble in water, they can't, unlike sugars or amino acids, simply dissolve in blood and be moved about, they need to be transported by carriers. These carriers differ, depending on where the triglycerides have immediately come from. When fat has just come from a meal, across the gut wall and into the blood, the triglycerides are transported as chylomicrons. Chylomicrons and their cargo of triglycerides have two primary destinations, either to be delivered directly as fuel to the muscles, or to be sent to the fat cells for storage. Both muscle and fat cells have lipases on their surface that recognise chylomicrons, allowing them to 'dock' to the cell. These same lipases then remove the fatty acids from the glycerol backbone, all while still on the cell surface, resulting in 'free' fatty acids, which then get absorbed by the cell. In fat cells, the free fatty acids and glycerol are reassembled to triglycerides, which is how they are stored. In muscles, however, once the fatty acids are absorbed into the cell, they are not stored but put to use immediately, generating ATP. Most cells can't, however, recognise and extract fatty acids from chylomicrons; rather, they use fatty acids that are actually released from fat. In fat cells, otherwise called adipocytes, when the body's energy levels are low, the enzyme 'hormone-sensitive lipase' gets activated, which converts triglycerides into free fatty acids. These free fatty acids are then released into the bloodstream where they bind to a carrier protein called albumin, and then get transported to all cells (including muscle cells) that need them as fuel.

The bottom line is that a typical molecule of fatty acid produces a total of 106 ATP when metabolised in the presence of oxygen.

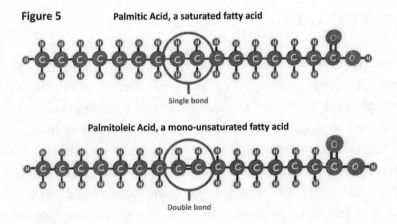

Figure 5　　**Palmitic Acid, a saturated fatty acid**

Single bond

Palmitoleic Acid, a mono-unsaturated fatty acid

Double bond

A typical fatty acid would be palmitic acid, which is the most common saturated fatty acid found in plants and animals. If you look at the figure, all fatty acids have on one end a structure composed of one carbon (C), two oxygens (O) and a hydrogen (H), this is then followed by a long chain of carbons and hydrogens (hydrocarbons) of varying length. Palmitic acid has a chain of sixteen carbons, lauric acid has a twelve-carbon chain, oleic acid has an eighteen-carbon chain, etc. This hydrocarbon chain is the critical part of all fatty acids; it is where the energy is stored, ready to be extracted. And what is it that makes a fatty acid saturated or unsaturated? Well, most atoms can interact with another atom, and, depending on the number of electrons a given atom has, it can interact with more than one atom. For example, hydrogen can only interact with one other atom, oxygen can interact with two, while carbon, by its nature, can interact with up to four other atoms. If you look at the figure of the two different fatty acids, every interaction between atoms is indicated with a line. You can see that oxygen can interact with a carbon and a hydrogen, or it can even interact twice with the same carbon (this is known as a double bond and is represented by two lines). To determine if a fatty acid is saturated or unsaturated, you need to look at the hydrocarbon chain. A saturated fatty acid such as palmitic acid has single bonds all along the hydrocarbon chain, meaning that each carbon is interacting with four other individual atoms. If you look at palmitoleic acid, however, you will see that the middle two carbons are each missing a hydrogen atom, and instead there is a double bond between them. Palmitoleic acid is therefore a mono-unsaturated fatty acid, meaning there is one double bond in the hydrocarbon chain. If there is more than one double bond it then becomes a poly-unsaturated fatty acid.

In muscle cells, fatty acids are sent to the mitochondria and oxidised to make ATP, in a process called 'β-oxidation'. Because of the long hydrocarbon chains, β-oxidation of fatty acids is by necessity a step-wise process that removes two carbons from the hydrocarbon chain at a time, with each round producing one NADH, one $FADH_2$ and one acetyl-CoA. Acetyl-CoA then enters the Krebs cycle to produce an additional $FADH_2$ and three NADH. Oxidation of palmitic acid, which has sixteen carbons, would therefore take seven rounds of β-oxidation, producing seven $FADH_2$, seven NADH and eight acetyl-CoA. The eight acetyl-CoA, through the Krebs cycle, yields twenty-four NADH and eight $FADH_2$. Amazingly, the whole process is super-efficient, costing only two ATP. Once all of the NADH and $FADH_2$ is used to power oxidative phosphorylation, then the complete oxidation of one palmitic acid molecule would generate a net total of 106 ATP! Fat is like petrol or diesel, and other hydrocarbon fuels, in that it is so very energy dense. In fact, you can set fat on fire, just like oil or kerosene, and it would burn for a long time.

PROTEIN METABOLISM

Finally, we have the most complex of the three macronutrients to deal with, protein. Protein is complex for two major reasons.

First, unlike fat or carbohydrate, which are composed entirely of differing proportions and configurations of carbon, hydrogen and oxygen, protein contains (in addition to C, H and O) a significant amount of nitrogen. While the human body can store C, H and O or pretty much oxidise it completely, any nitrogen that is not used (as part of protein) has to be excreted.

Second, the building blocks of protein, amino acids, are not homogenous. While we consume a great variety of carbohydrates, once the vast majority are digested down, they end up entering the bloodstream as glucose. As for fat, while there are varying lengths and saturation of fatty acids, they are all hydrocarbon chains that are broken down by β-oxidation. Amino acids, however, come in twenty different varieties (twenty-two if you count 'atypical' amino acids), and they all require slightly different strategies to break down.

The first step in amino-acid metabolism is the removal of the 'amino' group, which is the part of the amino acid that contains the nitrogen. The 'amino' group is converted to ammonia, which is then transported to the liver where it is incorporated into urea and released into the blood. The kidneys then extract the urea from the blood, where it moves to the bladder and is excreted as urine. The second step is where the breakdown strategies of the different amino acids differ. For the purposes of metabolism, amino acids can be divided into two broad groups. Most amino acids can be considered 'glucogenic', meaning that once the amino group has been jettisoned, the remaining carbon backbone can enter into the Krebs cycle at different points, depending on the structure of the original amino acid. A few of the amino acids, however, are 'ketogenic', meaning they are converted first into ketone bodies (see page 92) before being metabolised. Many of you would have heard about the 'Keto' Diet, and it is from this word 'ketogenic' that the diet obtained its name. I discuss the Keto Diet in detail in Chapter 5.

YOUR SAVINGS ACCOUNT

After you eat, as the food is digested by your food-to-poop tube, the nutrients pass through the gut wall, and your blood glucose levels will rise. This rise in blood glucose is sensed by the pancreas, which then secretes insulin into the bloodstream. The increase in insulin triggers your muscles and fat, in particular, to absorb huge amounts of glucose, which is then metabolised to produce ATP. But what happens to the glucose that is not used immediately? It is stored as glycogen, primarily in the muscles and the liver. Glycogen is, like starch, made up of chains of glucose, but in a less linear and far more branched-out fashion: imagine the branches of a large oak tree, which is kind of what it looks like. Glycogen is an energy reserve that can be mobilised quickly to meet a sudden need for glucose. However, while the energy from glycogen is easily accessible, these chains of glucose are not a particularly efficient storage system. The problem is, to form 1 gram of glycogen you need 3 grams of water, thus there will always be an upper limit to the amount of glycogen you can store, as it is so bulky. Skeletal muscle can maximally store about 400 grams of glycogen and the liver stores about 90 to 110 grams. Throw in the 4 grams (plus or minus a gram or so, depending on when you last ate) of glucose that is circulating in your blood, and all of this equates to – using the Atwater factor of 4 calories per gram of carb – about 2000 calories of carbohydrates that your body is capable of storing; probably about a day's worth.

How about the fatty acids that you don't use immediately? These are, of course, sent to the fat cells, where they are converted to and stored as triglycerides. Here's the thing, fat contains no water at all (fat and water don't mix, after all) and is therefore energetically very dense. An average-size adult of healthy weight has between 10 and 20 kilograms of fat stores (ranging from a six-pack to love handles). Once again, using the Atwater factor of 9 calories per gram of fat, that equates to between 90,000 and 180,000 calories! If you assume that the average person requires 2000 to 2500 calories a day in order to survive, then 180,000 calories from your fat stores would be enough to keep you alive (although not comfortably) for between seventy-two and ninety days, nearly three months!

That leaves us with amino acids. We require a large amount of amino acids every day to maintain and repair our muscles and organs. The problem is, we cannot actually store anything beyond what we need immediately. There is no reservoir of spare amino acids hanging about to be used, just in case we get caught short. Anything not used, after the nitrogen-containing amino group has been removed, is then fed into the Krebs cycle, either directly or via metabolism of ketones, to form acetyl-CoA. If there is too much acetyl-CoA, it gets converted by the process of fatty-acid synthesis (the reverse of β-oxidation) into fatty acids, which are transported back to the fat cells to be stored. Incidentally, this is also what happens to excess glucose, after all of the glycogen stores have been filled. Spare glucose is broken down by glycolysis to pyruvate, converted to acetyl-CoA, synthesized into fatty acids, and then stored as fat. Thus, all excess energy, regardless of whether it is in the form of glucose, fatty acids or amino acids, is stored as fat. Fat, as you can clearly see, is our primary fuel store.

And this whole process of intermediary metabolism or fuel storage is controlled by insulin. The headline function of insulin is its role in controlling blood glucose levels, but actually, insulin flips the switch between storage or metabolism of all fuels. So, after a meal, high glucose levels mean high insulin levels, which in turn trigger glucose uptake into muscle and fat, and the conversion of glucose to glycogen in muscle and the liver. High insulin levels also push amino acids into the building of muscle (which is why insulin is known as an anabolic hormone) and acetyl-CoA into fatty-acid synthesis. Whereas low insulin levels mean low glucose levels, which then trigger the breakdown of glycogen into glucose to be released into the blood. Low glucose also triggers the breakdown of protein into amino acids, and the conversion of fatty acids into acetyl-CoA by β-oxidation.

DIFFERENT ORGANS NEED DIFFERENT FUELS

Some of the pathways I've spoken about are universal, in that they take place in every cell. Glycolysis is such an example. The Krebs cycle and oxidative phosphorylation are also universal, at least in every cell that has mitochondria. Here, our red blood cells are the exception, because they have no mitochondria, and so rely solely on glycolysis for energy. Then there are pathways that are organ specific. So, for example, gluconeogenesis takes place largely within the liver and kidneys, but never in muscle; and while fatty acids are used as fuel by most organs, the brain uses mostly glucose, and ketones in times of starvation. Here are some of the key organs and the fuels they use:

Brain. Our brain does not use fatty acids for fuel. Instead, it requires a steady supply of glucose. It is only 2 to 3 per cent of our bodyweight, but ends up using more than 25 per cent of the circulating glucose. Although, if necessary, such as during starvation, up to 50 per cent of its fuel requirements can be met by ketone bodies (see page 92).

Muscle. The major fuels utilised by our muscles are glucose (derived from glycogen), fatty acids, and ketone bodies. Our muscles can store glycogen, but can neither export glucose nor perform gluconeogenesis, as they haven't got the enzymes.

Heart. The heart is also a type of muscle, but one that works continuously and relies entirely on aerobic metabolism. When an individual is resting, the favoured heart fuel is fatty acids; although ketone bodies, lactate, pyruvate and glucose are welcome too.

Liver. Our liver sits at the crossroads for metabolism. Intermediary fuels coming from our diet are transported here first. It acts as a buffer of blood glucose, either through the breakdown of glycogen or, crucially, through gluconeogenesis. The liver can either synthesise or break down triglycerides, depending on demand for metabolic fuels. It is the key manufacturer of ketone bodies, but these are strictly for export to other organs; the liver does not have the required enzyme to use ketones as fuel.

Fat. Our fat or adipose tissue stores and releases fatty acids according to demand. Fat also releases hormones that regulate metabolism.

Pancreas. Blood glucose levels are sensed by the pancreas, which then releases insulin in response.

Kidneys. Our kidneys dispose of urea in urine, maintain the pH of our blood, and, like the liver, carry out gluconeogenesis (although as a minor partner), which is important during starvation (see below).

STARVATION

Now, everything I have detailed in this chapter thus far is what happens between our two to three meals a day, part of the 'normal' (such as it is) cycle of modern daily living. What happens, however, when things go south? What happens, for example, should we enter a period of starvation? I am not referring here to our common use of the term, such as in the following sentence,

'Gosh, I'm starving tonight! I really fancy fish and chips ... I might get a large portion of chips!'

I am referring here to locusts and famine, actual biblical starvation; nearly non-existent in today's developed world, of course, but a reality for our ancestors tens of thousands of years back. Starvation is therefore a scenario we would have been able to adapt to, at least temporarily, otherwise we wouldn't be here now. Given that there are only enough carbohydrate stores in our body to last about a day, one of the key metabolic adaptations to starvation in many tissues in our body, particularly our muscles, is to shift to burning fat. This is to ensure that whatever glucose is left is reserved for the brain, since, as established above, the brain cannot metabolise fatty acids; its primary fuel is glucose. This is because our brain does all the command and control, so it needs to still be able to put together a cogent strategy to track down food, even in a haze of hunger. The second key metabolic adaptation is that the liver really ramps up gluconeogenesis (remember 'new glucose formation' as opposed to glucose obtained from glycogen stores) to ensure that blood glucose levels remain nearly constant. After forty hours of fasting nearly all of the glucose coming from the liver will have been generated from gluconeogenesis.

KETONES

In most tissues and organs, all (or certainly the vast majority of) acetyl-CoA enters the Krebs cycle, going on to then generate ATP. In the liver, however, under a number of different conditions, such as during fasting, starvation, a low-carbohydrate diet or prolonged strenuous exercise, a significant fraction of acetyl-CoA is converted by a process called ketogenesis to ketone bodies, or simply ketones (Figure 6). Another metabolic adaptation of starvation is the use of ketone bodies as a key fuel. These ketones are transported to other tissues, particularly to muscles, the heart and the brain, where they are used as an alternative source of fuel. Once ketones reach their destination, they are converted back to acetyl-CoA, and then used to generate energy.

Figure 6

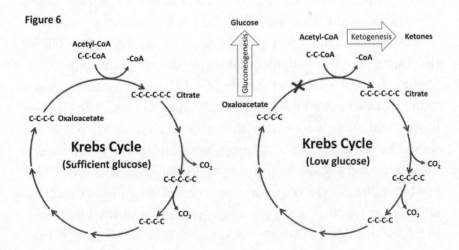

Why does this happen?

It has a lot to do with the Krebs-cycle intermediate oxaloacetate, which if you recall starts off the Krebs cycle by reacting with acetyl-CoA. Oxaloacetate also happens to be in the gluconeo-genesis pathway, in which pyruvate is converted into glucose; the first step of this conversion is pyruvate being converted into oxaloacetate. Why am I telling you any of this? Well, in starvation, a low-carbohydrate diet or prolonged strenuous exercise, all of the glycogen stores would have been used up, and there is therefore very little glucose available. The liver's response is to use gluconeogenesis to maintain blood glucose levels. Thus any oxaloacetate that is hanging about will be preferentially shunted into gluconeogenesis. If there is not enough oxaloacetate around, then the Krebs cycle begins to slow down, resulting in a build-up of acetyl-CoA (Figure 6). Something else that happens in starvation or a low-carbohydrate diet is that the body primarily burns fat for energy, because there is very little in the way of carbohydrates around. When fatty acids are metabolised by β-oxidation, this creates more acetyl-CoA, which is then converted, by ketogenesis, to ketones that are released by the liver into the blood. All cells with mitochondria can then take up these ketones, which are converted back into acetyl-CoA and used as fuel. No other tissue can divert its oxaloacetate into the gluconeogenic pathway in the way the liver does.

In starvation, you not only burn fat, but you also begin to lose muscle mass, that is, you begin to break down protein. The breakdown products of amino acids feed into the Krebs cycle, eventually ending up as either oxaloacetate (which supplies gluconeogenesis), or acetyl-CoA (which ends up as ketone bodies).

TYPE 1 DIABETES

Type 1 diabetes Mellitus, or simply type 1 diabetes, is an auto-immune condition where the body's immune system attacks and destroys the pancreas, and, critically, its ability to produce any insulin.

Because insulin plays a central role in controlling intermediary metabolism, diabetes ends up wreaking havoc on almost all metabolic pathways. Without insulin, muscle and fat cannot take up glucose from the blood after a meal, and glycogen will not form in the liver. As a consequence, blood glucose levels become so elevated that the glucose spills over into the urine. This results in more water being drawn into the bladder to try to dilute out the glucose. In fact, *diabētēs* (from Greek) means 'one that straddles', or specifically 'a siphon', which gave rise to the use of *diabētēs* as the name for a disease involving the discharge of excessive amounts of urine. Diabetes was first recorded in English, in the form *diabete*, in a medical text written around 1425. In 1675, Thomas Willis added the word *mellitus*, from the Latin meaning 'honey', a reference to the sweet taste of the urine. This sweet taste had been noticed in urine by the ancient Greeks, Chinese, Egyptians, Indians and Persians.

In addition to promoting glucose uptake and glycogen formation, insulin also pushes amino acids into the building of muscle and acetyl-CoA into fatty-acid synthesis. In the absence of insulin, everything is reversed, resulting in an uncontrolled breakdown of fatty acids and eventually muscle protein. This is why diabetes has been famously described as 'starvation in the midst of plenty', because without insulin, all of the intermediary nutrients of glucose, fatty acids and amino acids cannot be harnessed effectively.

Another prominent characteristic of uncontrolled diabetes is 'diabetic ketoacidosis'. With no glucose getting into cells coupled with a rapid breakdown of both fatty acids and amino acids, huge amounts of ketone bodies are formed and secreted into the bloodstream. Why is this dangerous? The issue here is not with the ketones *per se*, but with the fact that the ketones are acidic. Our blood pH is tightly regulated between 7.35 and 7.45. The pH scale goes from 0 to 14, indicating how acidic or alkaline a solution is. The middle of the scale is 7, which is neutral. Any number below that is acidic and any number above 7 is alkaline. Our blood is therefore slightly alkali. When it is suddenly flooded with a large amount of ketones, the blood begins to acidify. The moment the blood pH drops to between 7.0 and 7.25, drowsiness begins to set in. Once you go below pH 7.0, you could end up in a coma, and if the problem is not fixed rapidly, death follows quickly. So ketoacidosis is not a good situation to be in.

Before 1922, type 1 diabetes was a death sentence. There would be these horrific wards set up where diabetics, many of them children, would simply waste away, as if dying of starvation. Nutrients were being consumed, but would just run right through the body. Most patients would be in a diabetic coma by the time death took them. Then, in 1922, Sir Frederick Grant Banting and Charles Herbert Best, in the lab of J.J.R. Macleod in Toronto, discovered insulin. Michael Bliss wrote in the introduction to his remarkable book *The Discovery of Insulin*: 'Those who watched the first starved, sometimes comatose, diabetics receive insulin and return to life saw one of the genuine miracles of modern medicine.'[5]

Banting and Macleod won the Nobel Prize in Physiology or Medicine for its discovery in 1923.[6]

WHAT DO WE USE ALL THIS ENERGY FOR?

In this chapter, I've gone into quite some detail about how we extract energy from food: how we first digest it into its constituent parts, and then how our body painstakingly uses these intermediaries to generate ATP, the energy currency of life on Earth. I don't deny that many elements have been quite complicated; they still are to me, and I teach it every year to first-year medical and veterinary students! But I hope that the general concepts, which are what are important, were clear.

However, let's take another look at the final part of the equation we have been exploring over these first three chapters:

C – The number of usable calories we finally get out of the food.

While I have now explained how we get the calories out of food, we still have to work out how many of these calories are actually usable. In order to figure that out, we first need to understand what exactly we use the energy we extract from food for. And for that, we need to proceed to Chapter 4.

CHAPTER 4

What do we use energy for?

'When the spirits are low, when the day appears dark, when work becomes monotonous, when hope hardly seems worth having, just mount a bicycle and go out for a spin down the road, without thought on anything but the ride you are taking.'

Sir Arthur Conan Doyle 1896, in *Scientific American*

The small alpine town of Bourg D'Oisans, at the base of the ski station of L'Alpe d'Huez, can best be described as a cycling Mecca. In the summer months, cyclists from all over the world converge on this little town to climb any number of mountain passes and ski stations in the area. La Marmotte is an annual cyclosportive that begins from Bourg D'Oisans and takes in three of the most famous mountains in the area: the Col du Glandon, the Col du Galibier and the mythical twenty-one hairpin bends up to L'Alpe d'Huez, giving a distance of 174 kilometres (110 miles) and 5000 vertical metres (17,000 feet) of climbing. In 2006, Nick Jarvis, who was best man at my wedding, agreed to tackle this madness with me.

We arrived in Bourg D'Oisans a couple of days before to acclimatise and register for the ride. Would you believe, though, that ride registration was at the TOP of L'Alpe d'Huez?! The organisers clearly had a perverse sense of humour. So on Thursday, with our bikes out of their cases and built up, we strapped on our gear and headed to the base of the Alpe. The climb up L'Alpe d'Huez was first used by the Tour de France in 1952 and has been used at least every other year since. Because it is almost always placed at the end of a stage, it has been the scene of many a famous and dramatic victory. Each of the twenty-one bends is numbered in reverse and each is named after a rider who has won at the top of the Alpe. As we made our way up the 10 per cent gradient at the start of the climb to bend twenty-one, I looked up at the name on the sign . . . 'Lance Armstrong'!! I must point out that this was in 2006, long before his dramatic fall from grace in 2012, but I did look it up recently, and while Armstrong's seven Tour de France victories have since been stripped from him for 'pharmaceutically assisted' cycling, his name still adorns bend twenty-one of L'Alpe d'Huez.

The 15 kilometre (9 mile) climb from Bourg (altitude 719 metres; 2358 feet) up to 1880 metres (6167 feet) took us eighty minutes (the professionals would have done it in half the time). At the top, I felt a little tired but otherwise I thought to myself, 'Hey! This is going to be all right!' What a fool!

The morning of the race, Nick and I arrived at the starting area in Bourg town centre at 6.45 a.m. It was only then that we realised the scale of this event . . . there were over eight thousand registered riders! We were organised NOT by ability (like the London marathon) but by our dossard number. I was number 2042 and Nick was 2068, so we were toward the front of the bunch. Just take a moment to imagine over eight thousand cyclists on narrow streets in a French village . . . the group must have stretched back nearly a mile! And, whooo, boy, those machines! If you are into your cycling, it was like 'bike-porn'. Never had I seen so much expensive carbon fibre in such a small patch of real estate. Although most of the riders were of European extraction (the Dutch and French were probably in the overwhelming majority), there were riders from every corner of the globe. Ninety per cent of the riders were male (M.A.M.I.L.s, middle-aged men in Lycra . . .) and EVERYONE looked skinnier and fitter than me . . . I was beginning to get very nervous.

Seven thirty a.m. arrived and before we knew it WE WERE OFF!! The first few miles of the course were flat and, because we were cycling with so many other riders in a peloton-type situation, there was no wind resistance and we were coasting along at over forty kilometres per hour (twenty-five miles per hour) with almost no effort. We passed through the village of Allemont (820 metres; 2690 feet) and then UP we went for our first big climb of the day, to the Col du Glandon. Very quickly, the peloton began to string out as riders found their ability; there is nowhere to hide on the side of a mountain. A road sign helpfully informed us '25 kilometres (16 miles) to the summit'. I shifted to a low gear, settled into a rhythm and started spinning. As we passed through several small mountain villages, the residents would cheer from the roadside or their balconies, '*Allez! Allez!*'. Otherwise, all around was the sound of breathing, the shifting of gears, metal on metal, chain on cogs, tyres on tarmac, and, when you caught the wind in the wrong direction, the sometimes overwhelming odour of sweaty Lycra. There was not a lot of talking any more.

One hour into the climb and I realised that I had grossly underestimated the difficulty and length of this first mountain. How could I possibly be quite this tired so early on in the race? Signs continued appearing at regular intervals on the side of the road, '10 kilometres to the summit', '8 kilometres', 6, 4, 2, 1 . . . It took another hour to get up the Col du Glandon (1924 metres; 6312 feet). We got to the top and stopped for a breather. Twenty-two miles into this ride, with a climb *twice this size* yet to come and my legs already felt like jelly.

The summit of the Glandon was supposed to bring welcome relief in the form of food and water. However, there appeared to be an almighty scrum of riders trying to get off the mountain. As we searched for news, it emerged that there had been a horrible accident involving a number of riders on the descent and it was serious enough for the race to be paused while four ambulances and medics on motorbikes went down to clear things up. Because we had arrived thirty minutes into the stoppage, the summit was already packed like sardines, and there was no way we could move to find food. I pulled out one of the energy bars that I had with me and settled down to wait. As I was munching, I looked at the back of the pack. This was an oat and blueberry energy bar. Vital statistics: 68 grams, 268 calories; 5.2 grams fat, 44 grams carbs (with 22 grams sugar), 9.4 grams protein, and 4 grams fibre. Food of the gods, clearly.

An hour later, we were finally let past the police blockade twenty riders at a time, we were cautioned to take it easy, and down we went. It soon became obvious why so many accidents occur on this descent off the Glandon. First, the initial few miles of hairpin bends were steep and narrow with NO protective barrier between rider and oblivion. If you simply let go of your brakes, you would touch fifty miles per hour without peddling. You then needed to slow down to ten miles per hour to make each of the bends safely (I was NOT going anywhere near the edge of the road . . .) With all that braking, you could feel the heat coming of the wheel rims. Second, amazingly, the roads remained opened . . . so you also had to contend with the (admittedly light) traffic. All in all, this was a potent brew for a spectacular accident if you needed to sneeze or scratch your nose at the wrong time.

As we dropped down the mountain, the air temperature rose steadily so that by the time we hit the low-point (altitude-wise) of the ride, the little village of Sainte Marie de Cuines (420 metres; 1378 feet), it was eleven a.m. and a muggy 33°C. We cycled in the valley for fifteen miles or so and before we knew it, it was time to start climbing again, up to the Col du Télégraphe (1570 metres; 5151 feet) and then further beyond that, the giant Col du Galibier (2642 metres; 8668 feet). This next test was really one BIG climb, punctuated only by a five-minute descent into Valloire (1430 metres; 4691 feet) from the Télégraphe.

This was where Nick and I made a crucial rookie error. The climb up the Télégraphe was being done in the midday sun, both Nick and I were down to one full bottle of water each, and the only food we had taken on board since breakfast was that energy bar at the top of the Glandon. At the base of the climb, there was a crowded little corner shop, carbon fibre scattered all around the entrance, with a queue of riders waiting to get in. After surveying the scene we, foolishly as it transpires, elected not to stop for water or food, opting instead to fill up at the free food stop on the top of the Télégraphe. The climb was supposed to take a little over an hour ... we were fifty miles and one mountain into the ride, so naturally feeling a little tired and maybe a tad hungry, surely we were going to be fine.

Nope. Not even close.

I ran out of water halfway up the climb, at which time the heat was rising inexorably (it felt like 35°C now) and the sun was at its strongest. Then that awful feeling crept up, slowly at first, then suddenly like I'd slammed against a wall. I started to get 'the knock', the cyclist term for when you get serious hunger wobbles. I had a couple of pouches of those sickly energy gels, pure sugar in effect, which I tried to squeeze into my mouth. I was so hungry that the first one missed, squirting sticky syrup across my face and onto my jersey (marvellous, just what I needed). I got the second pouch on target and I swallowed the syrup, but aside from making me feel nauseous, it did nothing to quell the wobbly feeling. The problem is, once you get 'the knock', it is very difficult to come back from it. I slowed down to an absolute crawl, and felt simply awful. We had just got to the halfway point as well. Fifty-five miles done, fifty-five miles to go; halfway there, living on a prayer, sang someone once. How on earth was I going to finish? What a disaster.

'The knock' or 'hitting the wall' (in running parlance) occurs when you have used up your carbohydrate energy reserves – glycogen – in the midst of an endurance activity. However, I was clearly still carrying copious amounts of stored energy on myself in the form of fat. So how come I couldn't use those 'fat calories' instead? What is special about 'carb calories'?

ENERGY EXPENDITURE

OK, so all that painstaking effort we go through to carefully extract energy from food in order to make that body-weight's worth of ATP we go through every day, what do we use it for, exactly? Well, everything really; walking, running, sleeping, thinking, reproducing, eating, digesting, talking, yelling, singing, swimming, cycling, shivering, living . . . everything.

Our energy expenditure can be, broadly speaking, divided into three major components: 1) basal metabolic activity, which is the energy associated with maintaining all of the major body functions while at rest, and constitutes the largest proportion of daily energy expenditure, between 60 and 75 per cent; 2) physical activity, which covers energy expended due to any muscular activity, including shivering and fidgeting, as well as exercise for the sake of exercising, and constitutes 15 to 30 per cent of daily expenditure; and 3) diet-induced 'thermogenesis', which is the energy, in heat, that is given off after we have eaten, and constitutes approximately 10 per cent of daily energy expenditure.

1. Basal metabolic rate

The scientific definition of 'basal metabolic rate' or BMR is the amount of energy that a resting, fasted adult in a 'thermoneutral environment' is expending. Resting, because anything more than that would fall into the 'physical activity' category, and fasted, because when we eat we put out copious amounts of heat, as we will see later (see page 122). How about thermoneutral? Well, that is the temperature at which a healthy adult can maintain their normal body temperature without needing to use energy above and beyond basal metabolic rate; this is typically between 20°C and 30°C, depending on the size of the person and how much clothing, if any, they have on.

Thus, this basal metabolic rate is, in effect, the minimal amount of energy required for life. It is to make sure that even when sleeping, all of our organs are functioning; that we are breathing and our heart is beating, that our brain works, that our liver and kidneys continue to detox our blood, that our immune system continues scanning for infection, etc. etc. Yet, in spite of it just being enough energy for life support, BMR still takes up the lion's share of our quota of ATP, accounting for anywhere between 60 and 75 per cent of daily energy expenditure. And on top of that, this is the energy expenditure component that we have least control over . . . in fact, we can actually do little to nothing about modulating our BMR. Although prolonged physical activity does increase BMR marginally and temporarily, the biggest influence on BMR is bodyweight, or to be more accurate, body size.

'The reason I am so large is because my metabolism is slow.' How often have you heard that, or even thought that about yourself? Many people think that skinny wiry-type folk must have an engine that is running faster, because they appear to be zipping about, to be more energetic, more agile, whereas larger people often seem slower, apparently weighed down by inertia, lumbering about. Nothing could be further from the truth. A tiny, old-school Mini Cooper might seem zippy and fast compared to a large lumbering 4×4 SUV, but the SUV will always have a higher fuel consumption than the Mini. The same is true for humans and metabolism. In fact, the same is true for all living creatures: the larger and heavier the body, the more fuel required to run it, the higher the metabolic rate.

Metabolism, however, does not have a linear relationship with weight. Meaning a person who is twice the weight of another does not have a BMR that is twice as fast. It was Max Rubner (of calories fame), during his time in Marburg, Germany in the 1880s, who devised the ingenious calorimetric methods required to work out the relationship between body size and BMR. Remember that it was Rubner who constructed the first self-recording whole-body calorimeter, and began using it to measure the metabolic rates of dogs. He demonstrated, for example, that the first law of thermodynamics (that energy can be neither created nor destroyed, just transformed) applied not only to inanimate machines such as steam engines, but to dogs, and hence other living organisms as well. Using this same equipment, he showed that the relationship between metabolic rate and body size was not with the weight of the animal, but rather with the surface area of the animal; Rubner's surface law.[1] Why would this be? Because the surface-area-to-volume ratio of an animal is critical to their rate of heat loss and hence their metabolic rate.

Animals are, of course, complex and non-uniform in their shape, which makes things more difficult to visualise, so let me use a simpler and more uniform shape as an illustration.

Imagine a cube, 1cm × 1cm × 1cm. The volume of the cube would therefore be $1 \times 1 \times 1 = 1cm^3$. Its surface area would be 1cm × 1cm for each side = $1cm^2$, × 6 sides = $6cm^2$. Thus the surface-area-to-volume ratio of this small 1cm cube is 6:1.

Now imagine a larger cube, 10cm × 10cm × 10cm. The volume of the cube would be $10 \times 10 \times 10 = 1000cm^3$, while its surface area would be 10cm x 10cm for each side = $100cm^2$, × 6 sides = $600cm^2$. The surface-area-to-volume ratio of this larger cube, equivalent in volume to, for example, a large rodent, is 600:1000, which simplifies to 3:5.

What if we jumped up another magnitude in size to a 100cm × 100cm × 100cm cube? Then, its volume would be $1,000,000cm^3$

(equivalent in volume perhaps to a large mammal such as a cow) and surface area 60,000cm^2, giving a surface-area-to-volume ratio of 60,000:1,000,000, which simplifies to 3:50.

Rubner's so-called 'surface law' states that the relative metabolic rate of a given animal decreased with the same rate as its surface-area-to-volume ratio. Put simply, the smaller the animal, the more surface area they will have in relation to their volume, and the more heat they would lose. Hence they would require a higher metabolic rate per gram of bodyweight in order to maintain body temperature, as compared to a larger animal. But a cow, which is roughly a thousand times larger than a rat, will always have a higher metabolic rate, just not a thousand-fold more. Rubner calculated that the metabolic rate of an animal increases approximately with its mass raised to the power of ⅔.

As you might imagine, however, life and biology was never going to be as neat and tidy as one little ⅔ exponent. In the 1930s, along came Max Kleiber, a Swiss agricultural biologist, who performed the same metabolic-rate experiments as Rubner but using a larger size range of living creatures. Kleiber did verify the principle of Rubner's 'surface law', but found that the metabolic rate of an animal increased approximately with its mass raised to the power of ¾.[2] This became known as Kleiber's law. Then began nearly a century of scientists arguing which exponent, Rubner's ⅔ or Kleiber's ¾, was better for describing the relationship between body size and metabolic rate.

But what did these exponents worked out by Rubner and Kleiber mean, exactly? Let's take for comparison a mouse weighing 25 grams and a cat weighing 2500 grams. The cat is therefore 100 times heavier than the mouse. In order to use Rubner's and Kleiber's exponents to calculate their difference in metabolic rate, you have to raise the weights of each animal to either the power of ⅔ or ¾. So:

Rubner's ⅔: Mouse, $25^{⅔} = 8.64$

Cat, $2500^{⅔} = 189.1$

$189.1 \div 8.64 = 21.7$

Kleiber's ¾: Mouse, $25^{¾} = 11.18$

Cat, $2500^{¾} = 353.6$

$353.6 \div 11.18 = 31.6$

If Rubner is correct, then a cat having a mass 100 times that of a mouse will use about 21.7 times the energy of the mouse, whereas if Kleiber is correct, then that same cat will consume 31.6 times the energy the mouse uses. In this particular example, it just so happens that Kleiber's ¾ better predicts the difference in metabolic rate between a cat and a mouse. However, Rubner's ⅔ is a better predictor for other animals. So, as with most things in life, it all depends.

Here's the bottom line: having a singular exponent to accurately predict the relationship between metabolic rate and mass of all living creatures would only work if all species were the same shape and of the same density, which is clearly not the case. Animals vary both in shape and density, influenced by the relative size of bones and fat content as well as, for example, the presence of air sacs in birds and air bladders in fish. But it doesn't change the crucial basic principle that the larger the animal, the higher the BMR. Although BMR is an artificial physiological construct that animals rarely show under natural conditions (no animal in the wild is going to be lying around waiting to have their BMR carefully measured, they'd be eaten pretty quickly), it remains an established benchmark for comparing metabolic intensity between species.

How do we measure BMR?

There have been a number of methods, some more than two hundred years old, developed to measure metabolic rate in living animals. There was the very first ice-calorimeter, built and used by

Antoine Lavoisier in the 1760s to measure the heat given off by a guinea pig; the self-recording calorimeter built by Rubner in the 1880s to measure the metabolic rate of dogs; and the Atwater–Rosa Calorimeter in the 1890s used to measure the metabolic rate of humans.[3] Today, the very best technology we have for measuring BMR still uses the same fundamental principles that were established by these pioneers.

There are two 'gold-standard' techniques in use today for the measurement of metabolic rate. The first is a high-tech spruced-up version of the original Atwater-Rosa design, a chamber calorimeter. These are hotel-room-sized chambers that are entirely sealed. Air going into and out of the room, including the amount of oxygen and carbon dioxide, can be controlled and measured. We breathe in oxygen as fuel and breathe out carbon dioxide as exhaust, so measuring the ins and outs of this process allows us to indirectly calculate energy expenditure. You have to live in the chamber calorimeter for a few days, during which your metabolic rate can be measured when you are resting, when you are eating and, if there is a stationary bike in the room, when you are exercising. But as you might imagine, such rooms are technologically very complex, and as such there are only a handful in the UK, for instance. So this method, although invaluable in a clinical or research setting, cannot be realistically scaled up to a population level.

The second technique involves the use of a substance called 'doubly labelled water'. The chemical formula for normal everyday water that we drink, take a shower in and swim in is, as we know, H_2O; consisting of two hydrogen atoms and one oxygen atom. The vast majority of hydrogen atoms are formed of a nucleus of one proton, which is positively charged, and one orbiting negatively charged electron. Many atoms, however, have different rare but naturally occurring versions that vary in their number of neutrons, known as isotopes. Because a neutron is neutral, carrying neither a positive or negative charge, aside from altering mass it changes little else about the characteristics of that particular atom. Some isotopes have an unstable ratio of neutrons to protons in their nucleus, causing them to 'decay', sending out sometimes damaging particles; these are known as radioactive isotopes. Other isotopes are, for some physics explanation that escapes me, stable, meaning that the proton-to-neutron ratio within the nucleus is at some sort of equilibrium and does not decay over time. This is true, for instance, for hydrogen, which has a stable isotope with an additional neutron in its nucleus called 'deuterium'. Because electrons weigh next to nothing, all of an atom's mass comes from the protons and neutrons (both of which weigh nearly the same) that form the nucleus. Thus deuterium, which has both a proton and a neutron in its nucleus, weighs about twice as much as regular hydrogen, so is also known as 'heavy hydrogen'. One in every 6420 or so hydrogen atoms is deuterium. As for oxygen atoms, most are formed of a nucleus of sixteen protons and sixteen neutrons, with sixteen orbiting electrons. But in about one out of every five hundred oxygen atoms, instead of sixteen neutrons there are eighteen neutrons in the nucleus. This is a stable isotope of oxygen called 'Oxygen-18' or '^{18}O'. 'Doubly labelled water' is H_2O that is made of deuterium and ^{18}O, therefore both the hydrogen and oxygen components of water are, in effect, 'labelled', hence the name. Doubly labelled water is denser than normal water, because deuterium and ^{18}O are both heavier than their more common counterparts, and is a whole lot more expensive than even the fanciest of bottled water (you are not going to see it at your local supermarket any time soon) because of the need to enrich for the rare isotopes, but it certainly looks like water, feels like water and, by all accounts, tastes like water.

Why is this weird boutique water useful in measuring metabolic rate? Because if one was to drink a known dose of doubly labelled water and hence a known dose of traceable heavy hydrogen and

^{18}O, you could then track what happens to these isotopes. Once drunk, this known amount of labelled H_2O is then diluted into the rest of the water in the body. As we discussed in Chapter 3, when we break down carbon-containing carbs and fat to release energy through the Krebs cycle, carbon dioxide, or CO_2, is released as a by-product. Carbon dioxide is formed of two oxygen atoms and only one carbon atom, but there are simply not enough oxygen atoms found in fat and carbs (which are mostly carbon and hydrogen) to make CO_2. It turns out that one of the two oxygen atoms in CO_2 has to come from H_2O, and if there just happened to be some labelled H_2O hanging about, then some of the CO_2 would contain ^{18}O. Now, the way the doubly labelled water method works is that while ^{18}O can leave the body in two ways, either exhaled as CO_2 or excreted as 'waste' water (primarily through urine, sweat and breath), deuterium ONLY leaves the body as water.

Here is the crucial concept to grasp to understand how this technique works: the amount of labelled water consumed, and hence the ratio of deuterium to ^{18}O, is fixed, so by measuring the amount of deuterium lost through our waste water over time, we will also know exactly how much total ^{18}O has been lost. If we then measure how much of ^{18}O is lost through the waste water, we can calculate how much ^{18}O is lost through CO_2. Since the body ONLY produces CO_2 by metabolism, then the amount of oxygen that has left the body as CO_2 tells us how much energy has been produced over a given period of time, which is the definition of 'metabolic rate'.

Unlike a chamber calorimeter, the doubly labelled water approach can measure 'free-living' energy expenditure. In other words, aside from coming into the lab to have samples of urine, blood or sweat collected, this method will measure actual energy expenditure over a period of up to fourteen days. You can't lie, you can't cheat! But in and of itself, you can't use it to measure BMR, which needs to be done when a person has not eaten for twelve hours, and is resting, but not actually asleep. Tough, I know! However, when used in conjunction with a spell in a chamber calorimeter, the two techniques become complementary, providing a full picture of someone's real-world energy expenditure as well as their BMR.

2. Physical activity

Next, we have physical activity, which accounts for anywhere between 15 and 30 per cent of daily energy expenditure, and is the element we have most control over. The term 'physical activity' tends to evoke images of pumping iron in a gym like Arnold Schwarzenegger, running at defenders with the ball at your feet channelling Ronaldo or Lionel Messi, punching a side of beef in a refrigerated room à la Rocky, or cycling up the side of a mountain like Lance Armstrong (before we all knew his physical activity was pharmaceutically assisted). Those, and many other sporty pursuits are, of course, all different types of physical activity. But physical activity actually encompasses so much more, as it includes all manner of conscious muscular-dependent movement. There are a number of muscular activities, such as your heart beating, breathing or peristalsis in the gastrointestinal tract, that go on constantly from the day we are born till the day we die, which we cannot consciously control. These are part of the life-support system and the energy required to run them forms the basal metabolic rate. But almost any time you use your skeletal muscles (muscles attached to and designed to move our skeleton) – wiggling your pinky finger as you are lying in bed, walking downstairs to the kitchen, gardening, taking out the garbage, grocery shopping, walking the dog – is considered physical activity; it doesn't just refer to sport and overt exercise.

Feel the burn

Now, depending on the type of physical activity being done, whether high-intensity for a short duration, low-intensity for a long duration, or anything in between, your body will end up using different types and blends of fuel to generate ATP.

For activities with the very shortest of durations, such as serving in tennis, or throwing a javelin, discus or shot put, your muscles will simply use up the ATP that is already there. There is, however, only enough ATP hanging around our muscle cells for maybe two to four seconds of activity. So once that is exhausted, your body begins to use a staged system to regenerate ATP from ADP.

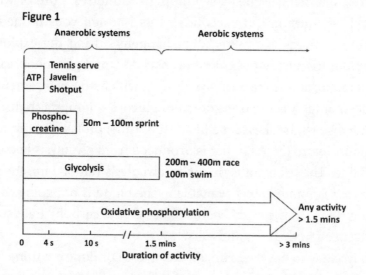

Figure 1

The first reserve is the 'phosphocreatine' system. During times of rest when there is an excess of ATP, a number of ATP are converted to ADP, with the phosphate group that is released in the process merging with a molecule called 'creatine', producing 'phosphocreatine', literally a creatine with a phosphate group attached. After the immediate local supplies of ATP are used up, the pool of phosphocreatine is activated and donates the phosphate group back to ADP, recharging it back up to ATP, ready to be used again. This gets us up to about eight- to ten-seconds' worth of activity; enough, for instance, to power Usain Bolt over 100 metres. For the 'phosphocreatine' system to be charged up again takes spare ATP, which means it takes a little bit of rest, or if you are really fit, a reduction in intensity of activity. At this point, Mr Bolt will do his 'superman' pose, and then head off to cool down, so his ATP levels are probably coming back up and his phosphocreatine system being recharged.

What happens in a 200-metre race, though, which someone like Usain Bolt or Dina Asher Smith or Alison Felix would run in around twenty seconds? Or Shaunae Miller-Uibo running 400 metres, or Michael Phelps swimming 100 metres, both of which would take around fifty seconds? This is when your immediate glucose reserves are used. What happens during the explosive, short-duration activities is that even as ATP and phosphocreatine are being used, the rate of glycolysis – which you will remember from Chapter 3 is the breakdown of glucose – jumps a thousand-fold. However, it takes just a little bit of time, probably around ten seconds before the ATP that is produced from glycolysis becomes available. The problem is that with glycolysis ramped up, the glucose that is immediately available in the blood is not going to last all that long, so the body begins to access the carbohydrate stores of glycogen in the liver and muscle.

Anyone who has ever run, swum, cycled or done anything hard for more than thirty seconds to a minute will know the burning sensation that builds up in the relevant muscle group that is being used. Glycolysis, which breaks each molecule of glucose down into two of pyruvate, is an anaerobic process, meaning it occurs in the absence of oxygen. This is advantageous because it can be mobilised very quickly, thus is appropriate for the powering of high-intensity and short bursts of activity. The problem, however, is that in the absence of oxygen, pyruvate gets converted to lactate and then to lactic acid, which is what causes the burning sensation in the muscles. In addition, glycolysis only produces a net gain of two ATP for each glucose molecule, which is not a great deal. Depending on how fit you are, anaerobic activity can be maintained for up to about ninety seconds. Then two things happen: first, the build-up of lactic acid becomes too painful for your muscles to function effectively . . . you can only 'feel the burn' for so long; and second, the energy requirements of the muscles surpasses what glycolysis is able to provide on its own. It is at this point that oxygen fully deploys, kicking off all of the aerobic processes.

'You are getting fitter!'

I have one of these heart-monitor things that you strap around your chest, which is linked via Bluetooth to an app and the GPS on my phone. I use it on my regular run, a five-mile loop through the country lanes and fields near my house, to track my speed and heart rate. Not that I am training for anything in particular; I just find it useful, as motivation more than anything, to relate how good or bad I felt during a given run to my average heart rate and how fast I actually completed the loop. The app also has a habit of chatting to me as I plod along. At every mile, for instance, I am informed by a female voice of my pace (minutes per mile) and my average heart rate. Most annoyingly, the voice will also periodically squawk 'You are burning fat!' or 'You are getting fitter!' – triggered, as far as I can tell, by whatever heart-rate 'zone' I happen to be entering. The app calculates what zone I'm in, based on what percentage of my 'maximal' heart rate I happen to be at. This is not, just to be clear, an empirical measure, which would have required me to be in a lab hooked up to breathing apparatus and cycling to exhaustion on a stationary bike. Rather, it is a 'back of the envelope' calculation that simply subtracts my current age from 220. At time of writing, I am forty-seven years old, which would make my estimated max heart rate 173 beats per minute. Given that the app tells me I spent nearly 20 per cent of my last run with my heart rate above 173 and

I certainly didn't feel faint or unwell, the '220 minus your age' max heart-rate estimation clearly leaves a lot of room for error. How fit and active someone is, whether they smoke or are pregnant and whether or not they are ill would all influence the actual max heart rate on any given day. Hopefully what this means is that I am fitter than the average forty-seven year old (I am ever the optimist)! Anyway, when my heart rate is above 70 per cent of my notional maximum of 173, which is 121 beats per minute, then the lady in the app tells me I am 'getting fitter'; whereas if I am working at a heart rate below 70 per cent of my maximum, then I am 'burning fat'.

The whole purpose of increasing heart rate during physical activity is to increase blood flow, and hence the delivery of oxygen throughout the body. Your skeletal muscles, and during a run they would of course be the large ones powering your legs, become like sponges, sucking in the oxygen from the blood. In the presence of oxygen, the conversion of pyruvate to lactate slows down, and pyruvate is, instead, preferentially broken down to acetyl-CoA. Acetyl-CoA is fed into the Krebs cycle, and then oxidative phosphorylation. This process of aerobic respiration parlays an additional twenty-eight ATP from pyruvate, which together with the two ATP produced through glycolysis means that each molecule of glucose yields thirty ATP. With that step up in energy supply, we are now in the realm of aerobic endurance activity.

In full aerobic flow, the other thing that happens is that the lactate that had initially built up from glycolysis, and continues to build up even during aerobic respiration, albeit more slowly, is cleared from the muscles into the bloodstream. One of the markers of 'fitness', in fact, is the speed at which you are able to clear lactate from your muscles; the quicker you can do that, the higher the intensity of activity (which increases lactate production) you can maintain over a longer period of time. An elite athlete will be very efficient indeed in clearing lactate from muscles, certainly when compared to a plodding chump like me! Once lactate is moved from the muscles and into the bloodstream, it is transported to the liver, where it is converted back to pyruvate and, through the process of 'gluconeogenesis' or new glucose formation (see Chapter 3), is transformed back to glucose. This 'new' glucose is shoveled back out into the bloodstream and taken back to the muscles to be used as fuel. This process is known as the Cori cycle, and during exercise, about 30 per cent of all glucose we use is derived from lactate 'recycling' to glucose.

However, the carbohydrate stores of glucose and glycogen will only last so long. When I head out on my typical weekend run, there will be, theoretically, enough glucose dissolved in my blood to power me for around four minutes. The body doesn't hang about waiting for all the blood glucose to be used before acting; instead, the moment my legs start working, the glycogen stores in my muscles begin to be broken down to glucose. At full capacity, muscles carry enough glycogen for roughly seventy minutes of activity. The glucose from muscle glycogen, however, is not secreted into the blood, but is produced exclusively for local use, to power just the muscles. The other organ with significant glycogen stores in the body is the liver. The liver holds enough glycogen for around twenty minutes of activity. These stores are broken down to maintain glucose levels in the blood. So all told, we hold enough carbohydrate stores for around ninety minutes of activity.

But, as we all know, our main long-term energy store is our fat. Taking away what we need to maintain our basal metabolic rate, we probably have enough fat stores to keep running for 4000 minutes or nearly three days straight! Assuming, of course, that we were not eating and we could maintain that level of activity ... theoretically possible, I guess, certainly 50,000 years ago on the Serengeti, but highly unlikely today.

Burning fat in the flames of carbohydrates

Fat is stored as triglycerides in our fat cells or adipocytes. When required, such as on a long run or cycle ride, hormone-sensitive lipase converts triglycerides into free fatty acids, which are then transported by albumin to the muscles. Within the muscle cells, the fatty acids are brought to the mitochondria where they are broken down by a process called β-oxidation (see Chapter 3), which produce acetyl-CoA, to feed into the Krebs cycle. While carbohydrates are almost immediately accessible, which is why they are preferentially used during explosive short-duration activities, fat is very energy dense and so is more appropriate to fuel endurance activities. β-oxidation of a typical fatty-acid molecule – palmitate, say – produces eight acetyl-CoA (compared to two acetyl-CoA for each glucose molecule), and therefore a whole heap of ATP. In fact, each molecule of palmitate produces a net of 106 ATP! That is nearly four times what each glucose molecule provides.

There is a common misconception that your body only begins to metabolise fat once all of the carbohydrate stores are used. In reality, while carbohydrates are indeed the fuel of choice during anaerobic activity, the moment all of your aerobic systems kick in, both fat and carbs are used. So the lady in my heart monitor is correct to inform me that I am 'burning fat', almost from the moment I begin my run. The issue is that because we have so many more fat stores than carb stores, the carbs will always run out first! Another thing that many don't know is that fat is actually oxidised more efficiently in the presence of carbohydrates. To understand why, we need to revisit the Krebs cycle.

Recall that the Krebs cycle is a controlled way of breaking carbon bonds to unlock the stored potential energy. The cycle 'begins' when acetyl-CoA is fed in, and the acetyl group, a two-carbon molecule, reacts with the four-carbon oxaloacetate, to form a six-carbon molecule citrate, which is why the Krebs cycle is also known as the 'citric-acid cycle'. Then follow a further nine steps, whereby citrate loses two of its six carbons, released as two molecules of carbon dioxide or CO_2, and is converted back to oxaloacetate, when another molecule of acetyl-CoA is fed in, and the cycle begins again. Oxaloacetate is normally replenished from within the Krebs cycle, but it can also be made from pyruvate, which, as we have discussed, comes from the breakdown of glucose by glycolysis. As you also know, pyruvate can be turned back into glucose by gluconeogenesis, and pyruvate being converted to oxaloacetate just so happens to be the first step in the process.

Figure 2

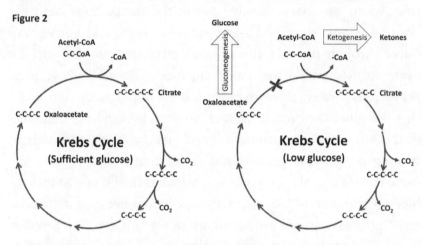

Why is this relevant? Under normal metabolic circumstances where there is ample glycogen storage to maintain circulating glucose at appropriate levels, oxaloacetate is readily available to combine with acetyl-CoA to power the Krebs cycle. If there is an increase in aerobic activity, more glucose and more fatty acids will be broken down, which means an increase in acetyl-CoA. Here is the important thing to understand: there needs to be enough oxaloacetate to react with the acetyl-CoA coming in from the breakdown of carbs and fat, otherwise the Krebs cycle begins to slow down. So under these circumstances of increased acetyl-CoA, some of the pyruvate, instead of being converted to acetyl-CoA, is converted to oxaloacetate, to make sure the Krebs cycle keeps on chugging along producing energy, and powering the muscles. Thus, while fatty acids provide most of the acetyl-CoA and therefore most of the ATP, the complete oxidation of fat happens most efficiently when there is enough glucose around to ensure sufficient oxaloacetate, hence the saying that 'fat burns in the flames of carbohydrates'.

What happens, however, if the physical activity you are participating in takes a really long time to complete? Such as perhaps cycling up the side of a mountain in France in the thirty-degree heat, where you have already been in the saddle more than five hours and you stupidly haven't eaten enough, and you've now burnt through the majority of your glycogen reserves, just for example? Remember that blood glucose levels always have to be preserved, because there are organs, most importantly your brain, that use glucose primarily as fuel. So your liver, whose main role in this situation is to maintain blood glucose levels, responds by turning on gluconeogenesis and converting both pyruvate and oxaloacetate to make 'new' glucose, which is then secreted into the blood. Oxidation of fatty acids also increases, because there is no more glycogen, hence producing more acetyl-CoA. The problem is, because oxaloacetate is now being shunted into gluconeogenesis, there is not enough of it to react with acetyl-CoA and the Krebs cycle begins to slow down. This is not an existential crisis, because the resulting build-up of acetyl-CoA is converted, by ketogenesis, to ketones that are released by the liver into the blood. All cells with mitochondria can then take up these ketones, which are then converted back into acetyl-CoA and used as fuel. The rate of ATP production is slower when relying on ketones, but the body, as always, is able to adapt.

Hitting the wall

The problem is, this adaptation takes time, and if your body is trying to adapt as you are, oh, I dunno, cycling up a big mountain, that is when you get 'the knock', the serious hunger wobbles. Marathon runners experiencing the equivalent phenomenon would call this 'hitting the wall'. And that was the dire situation I found myself in as I was trying to make it up the Col du Télégraphe on that hot summer's afternoon. Even though it was clear that I still had the vast majority of my fat reserves on board to be used (quick check just now . . . I can report it is all still there), the depletion of my glycogen reserves, those carbohydrate 'flames' to ensure efficient burning of fat, resulted in a sudden and precipitous slowdown of energy production. Experienced endurance athletes mitigate against this by first 'carbo loading' the night before to ensure their glycogen stores are filled to the brim (this I did, wolfing down the biggest portion of spaghetti I possibly had ever eaten), and eating carbohydrate-rich food, like energy bars, at regular intervals during the race itself to slow down the depletion of glycogen (this I did not do).

Anyway, Nick and I managed to just about make our way to the top of the Col du Télégraphe, taking us eighty minutes instead of the scheduled sixty minutes. Because of that stupid rookie feeding error, I expended a lot more energy than I had intended . . . energy I was going to need for the second half and MORE difficult part of the ride! Incidentally, I have never made that mistake again. Now, on long rides, I eat every hour, whether or not I feel hungry . . . in fact, if you feel hungry it probably is too late!

From the top of the Télégraphe we headed down the short descent into Valloire and the second official food stop. Actually before we got to the official stop, we noticed an enterprising business woman in a little shack on the side of the road selling *jambon et fromage* (ham and cheese) paninis and canned sodas. It looked all the world more appetising than the apples, soggy bread and disgusting isotonic drinks we were going to get up the road, so we stopped. It was the MOST lovely panini and the MOST lovely can of Coke in the world, and I felt better. We did stop to fill up our bottles with the puke-yellow isotonic drinks that, although sickly, would provide us with a valuable supply of sugar, and then we were climbing again.

The first couple of miles out of Valloire were surprisingly gentle, lulling us into a false sense of security. However, the gradient suddenly kicked up, hairpin bends started appearing and another helpful road sign informed us that there were 15 kilometres (9 miles) to the summit. The Col du Galibier is the **highest** mountain pass that is used by the Tour de France. As we ascended, the air became noticeably thinner, and as a result my breathing and heart rate increased to quite an uncomfortable level in order to bring enough oxygen to the mitochondria in the muscles, to power oxidative phosphorylation and generate ATP. And my legs, which were already suffering on the Glandon, felt like they were going to fail me at any point. It was horrendous and I wished it all to end immediately. However, even as the climb continued upwards (and I had the unfortunate experience of seeing the road rise up twisting and turning before me with seemingly no end) and I felt increasingly awful, I was still passing other cyclists, all of whom looked skinnier and fitter than me. Un-Christian-like though it was, the thought that these guys were actually feeling worse than me helped me eventually get to the top without giving up (barely).

We were now at 2642 metres (8668 feet) and 114 kilometres (71 miles) into the ride. The summit of the Galibier could not have been more than 6°C. Because were drenched in sweat from the climb, we started shivering the moment we stopped. So we pulled on our arm warmers and gilets, and began the superfast 48-kilometre (30-mile) descent back to Bourg D'Oisans and the base of the dreaded final climb up to L'Alpe d'Huez. This was without a doubt the best part of the whole day. The view (whenever it was safe for me to look), especially near the top, when we were actually higher than some of the glaciers, was simply spectacular.

The 30-mile descent from the top of Col du Galibier took just over an hour and we arrived at back in Bourg D'Oisans at the base of L'Alpe d'Huez at 5.30 p.m. It was now 160 kilometres (100 miles) into the ride. Including the one-hour delay at the top of Col du

Glandon, we had been on the road for ten hours. It was already the longest time I had EVER spent on a bike and I had another two hours to go! I ate a carbohydrate-rich energy bar (the flames to burn fat!), topped up my bottles and then began the final climb.

The day before the race, Nick and I were speaking to a nice Dutch couple who had (amazingly) started the ride six times (finishing five times). We asked them what the worst part of the ride was, and the guy pointed to L'Alpe. He said, 'When you get there at the end of the day, it is no longer cycling. It is surviving.' Hey, you know what? He was 100 per cent correct. I cranked my pedals at four to five miles per hour all the way to the top. On the way, helpful people gave me water (I was out and it was hot), poured cold water down my neck (a wonderful experience when you're on a bike and feel like you're dying) and a couple even gave me a helpful push.

As I entered the village of L'Alpe d'Huez proper, there was still 2 kilometres (1.2 miles) to go. But there were people cheering '*Allez! Allez!*' on the side, keeping me going. As I entered the finishing straight, I got out of the saddle and attempted to sprint (a loosely used term at this point in my day) for the finish. As I crossed the line, my electronic tag beeped and my time popped up, twelve hours for 174 kilometres and 5000 vertical metres. I was ecstatic that I didn't have to head upwards any more.

A reason to train

That ride nearly killed me. OK, that is clearly hyperbole, it didn't nearly kill me . . . but it certainly felt like it at points during the day. However, difficult as it might have been for me to imagine, I would have felt far worse, and in all probability would not have finished the ride, if I hadn't trained hard for six months before I got on the plane to France. In addition to my cycle commute of, at the time, twenty miles a day during the week, I would then get in a long ride of 50 to 70 miles on Sunday mornings.

What does training do? First, it improves aerobic fitness. This means increasing the volume of blood your heart can pump with each beat, making you able to function more comfortably at a higher heart rate, increasing the oxygen-carrying capacity of the blood, and improving the oxygen–carbon dioxide exchange in the lungs. Second, assuming you are training specifically for a particular event – running or cycling or swimming, or all three if you are training for a triathlon – it conditions the muscles for the task at hand. This improves the target muscle's size and strength, which for me would have been primarily the ones powering my legs, increasing the number of mitochondria per cell, and hence the amount of ATP produced per cell, as well as increasing the efficiency of lactate clearance from the muscles, so that they can operate at a higher intensity for longer.

A couple of things to consider, though. I live in Cambridge in the UK. For those of you who are not familiar with the area, this region is the flattest part of the whole UK, which makes training for an alpine cycling event a little tricky. I did go up and down my local hill (a two-minute climb at the most) multiple times (it got boring pretty quickly), and travelled to some of the hillier parts of the UK (Wales and the Lake District) for a couple of rides, but I would clearly have been in far better condition if I had lived in the Colorado Rockies or anywhere in the Alps. The other thing is that, while my personal biology, my genetics, will always limit the amount of improvement I am ever likely to achieve – I am never going to be Lance Armstrong, pharmaceutically assisted or not – I have never been as 'cycling fit' as I was back in 2006!

3. Diet-induced thermogenesis

Finally, we move to the third and smallest component of energy expenditure, that is 'diet-induced thermogenesis' (DIT), also known as the thermic effect of food. This is the amount of energy released, in heat, above the basal metabolic rate that results from the consumption of food, and accounts for around 10 per cent of daily expenditure.

It was Rubner, during his work on calorimetry, who in 1902 first noticed that the consumption of food stimulated heat production. Anecdotally, I know that I (like undoubtedly many of you) get a bit sweaty when I eat food, particularly when it is a big bowl of noodles in soup, for instance. That is, however, not DIT! Rather, it is because I am eating a big steaming bowl of soup!

There are, broadly speaking, two elements to DIT: there is an 'adaptive' component that serves to dissipate energy as heat when required, and there is the obligatory energy cost of digestion, absorption and assimilation of nutrients as well as the cost of synthesising body fat and protein, both of which are not mutually exclusive of each other. Critically, this is energy that is released from food that is, for want of a better term, 'lost'; it is neither stored nor used to generate ATP.

Thermogenesis

Thermogenesis literally means 'heat production'. This can occur as a result of physical activity – the actual contraction of skeletal muscles, either in the form of exercise or less obviously (or voluntarily) by shivering. This happens because the conversion of chemical energy (ATP) to mechanical energy (muscle activity) gives off heat.

However, thermogenesis also occurs independently of physical activity. We are warm-blooded, after all, and need to maintain our body temperature whether or not we are moving. ATP being converted to ADP is not always used to generate mechanical energy, for instance, but can go directly to producing heat. Another way of generating heat is through a process known as 'non-shivering' thermogenesis, and that happens at the level of the mitochondria, in certain tissues, including in brown fat and in our muscles. Brown fat is not fat, in that its main role is not to store triglycerides, rather it is brown-ish in colour because it is packed full of mitochondria, hence its name, and its primary role is to generate heat. The mitochondria function as cellular power stations, housing the processes of β-oxidation, the Krebs cycle and oxidative phosphorylation, thereby generating the vast majority of ATP. In oxidative phosphorylation, protons (H^+) are pumped from the matrix, across the inner mitochondrial membrane through to the intermembrane space, generating a positive electrical gradient, at which point the protons flow back into the matrix through ATP synthase, generating ATP. In brown fat, there is an 'uncoupling protein' that sits in the inner mitochondrial membrane that allows protons to leak from the intermembrane space back into the matrix, bypassing ATP synthase. It 'uncouples' the protons from the production of ATP, in the process generating heat.

Thus, food consumed in excess of immediate requirements, aside for being stored, can also be dissipated as heat when required, hence the term 'adaptive'. It can be considered as an energetically non-conservative mechanism that provides a form of output control in the regulation of energy balance.

The cost of doing business

Then there is the obligatory cost of doing business, the energy required for processing food for use and storage. This includes not only the energy expended to digest food, which is actually minimal, but all of the energy required to power intermediary metabolism as well. Whether or not you are moving glucose, fatty acids or amino acids into storage, or breaking them down into acetyl-CoA to generate ATP, there is an energetic cost. This 'diet-induced thermogenesis' actually lasts for a long time after the end of a meal, up to six hours, many studies have shown.

Because each of the different macronutrients take a different pathway before arriving at the common point of acetyl-CoA (see Chapter 3), each will have a different energetic cost, a different

DIT value. Fat is hugely energy dense, so while it may take seven rounds of β-oxidation to break down the fatty acid palmitate, for instance, that effort yields more than a hundred ATP molecules. It is a hugely efficient way of storing energy (which is why it is our primary way of storing energy) and hence its DIT value is between 0 and 3 per cent. When Atwater calculated the availability of calories, what he referred to as 'metabolisable calories' or the calories that have been digested and absorbed from the gut, his factor for fat was 9 calories per gram of fat. So if we now take into account the DIT value for fat, this means that for every 100 metabolisable calories of fat, it will cost between 0 and 3 calories to process. Thus the 'net metabolisable calories' for fat is nearly identical to Atwater's factor of 9 calories per gram.

Now, the DIT value for carbohydrates, depending on whether you use it immediately or store it first, is calculated to be between 5 and 10 per cent. This would mean that for every 100 metabolisable calories of carbs, it will cost between 5 and 10 calories to process. If we apply this DIT value to Atwater's carbohydrate factor of 4 calories per gram, that would make a 'net metabolisable' calorie factor of around 3.6 calories per gram of carb.

Then we get to protein, which has the highest thermic effect of all. The issue is the body has no protein storage capacity, so it requires immediate metabolic processing. While fat and carbs are each of broadly uniform structure and are therefore handled efficiently by the body, protein is an entirely more complex beast. Protein is not homogenous, but is instead made up of twenty structurally different building blocks known as amino acids, thus there are essentially twenty different metabolic pathways to get each amino acid to acetyl-CoA. On top of that, there is a requirement to extract the nitrogen from amino acids and to subsequently excrete it as urea. All of this has a high energy cost, which results in the production of a lot of heat. If you factor all of that in, then the DIT value for protein is anywhere from 15 to 30 per cent.

If we apply this to Atwater's protein factor of 4 calories per gram that would make a 'net metabolisable' calorie factor of between 2.8 and 3.4 calories per gram of protein. That is really quite a big difference.

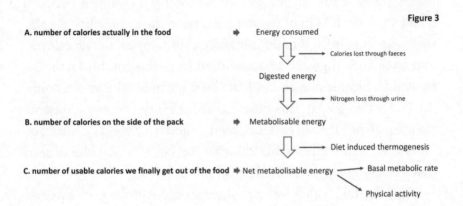

Figure 3

SO WHAT?

In Chapter 1 I charted the history of calorimetry and how the invention of bomb calorimetry allowed us to work out the total number of calories locked up in the food. In Chapter 2 I explored the work of Rubner and Atwater, and how they got us from the total number of calories in a food to the calorie-counts we see on most food packaging today. In the last two chapters, I have described how we convert the calories we eat into energy, what we use the energy for, and in doing so, explained why the calories on the side of the pack do not equate to the number of usable calories we finally get from food.

'So what?' you may well ask.

Well, you know all of those diets that we have all been on at one time or another? Those plans that reinvent themselves with a new mask and a new name come every January? Those approaches championed by Instagram gurus that, depending on the time of year, boost or detox or melt or cleanse or revitalise or heal <insert your favourite organ or biological process here>? As it turns out, this simple concept of 'caloric availability' explains how the vast majority of these diets that do actually work, work.

In the next three chapters, we move from the biochemistry of calorie metabolism to how different sources of calories actually influence our feeding behaviour. We will begin with understanding the power of protein. And to do that, we need to move on to Chapter 5.

CHAPTER 5

The power of protein

'When life gives you lemons, ask for something higher in protein'

Internet meme

I am based at the University of Cambridge and have been working on the genetics of obesity and how our brain controls food intake for more than twenty years now. Like all other jobs, there are pros and cons to being in this business. The biggest problem is that because most of us are, by definition, 'experts' at eating – knowing when, how much and what to eat, at least well enough to keep ourselves alive till now – most of us, therefore, have an opinion on eating, and by extension, many have an opinion about other people's weight. Having an opinion is not actually a negative per se, particularly if you keep it to yourself. It is when one's opinion tilts into being judgmental about somebody's body shape or size, and when it moves someone to begin imposing their way of eating on someone else, that it becomes an issue. So we now have the perennial problem of 'body-shaming' or 'food-shaming' others. It is interesting that while racism and sexism are no longer tolerated in large sectors of society (although I acknowledge we have a lot further to go), overtly judging someone's bodyweight is still considered acceptable by many, even amongst those who consider themselves 'socially enlightened'. While it is clear that the cause of obesity is a result of eating more than you burn – it is physics after all – it turns out that differences in our genetic make-up mean all of us behave differently around food. This is what I spend my time researching. Some of us, for instance, are slightly more hungry all the time and so eat more than others. Some of us might eat in response to stress, whereas others will stop eating as the result of that exact same stress. People who are overweight or are living with obesity are neither bad nor lazy; rather, they are fighting their biology. Bodyweight is not a choice. Trying to convince society otherwise, however, is like swimming upstream through treacle.

What this also means is that for folks who are carrying too much fat and need to lose weight, and there are many who do for the sake of their health, there is no magical one-size-fits-all solution. Any 'diet' that results in someone eating less is a diet that works. People say 95 per cent of diets don't work, but the truth is probably closer to the fact that 95 per cent of diets are impossible to stick to! Yet the diet industry is worth billions, with the 'eat like this and look like me' celebrities and Instagram 'health' gurus trading their wares, their 'effortless' solutions, on the basis of pseudoscience.

The positives of working in the field of obesity are many. For one thing, I love what I do and, if I am lucky enough, hope to continue doing this till the day I retire. How many people can say that, after all? Given that the global public health problem of obesity is not going away any time soon (this is not the positive part), it is actually entirely likely that I will be working in this space until I retire (this is the positive part). The topic of obesity and food intake is also very easy to engage others about (this is the positive 阳 yáng to the negative 阴 yīn above, with everyone having an opinion); it doesn't seem to matter if it is with other scientists, or with non-expert members of the public. For this reason, I have been privileged and fortunate to have had the opportunity to broadcast, write and speak on this subject over the years. But in keeping with the yīn & yáng theme, this public exposure also comes with its own challenges.

One recent December, Jane and I were at our friends Nick and Karen's place, in London, for a Christmas party. Jane and Karen were school friends and have known each other for decades, so this festive soirée was something of a fixture in our annual social calendar. On that particular December evening, with the party in full flow, Jane and I were hanging out in their slightly narrow but beautifully appointed kitchen, drinking (Jane with a glass of bubbles, naturally, and me a glass of 2017 Argentinian Malbec), canape-ing, and socialising like well brought-up guests. I struck up conversation with a gentleman whose wife was also a friend of Karen's. We were making drinks-and-nibbles type small-talk when Karen sashayed past, wearing a fabulous early twentieth-century 'flapper girl' outfit right out of *The Great Gatsby*, in her 'hostess with the mostest' role, saying:

'Oh good, you've met. John, did you know that Giles presents TV shows about diets? He's also just written a book on the subject as well!'

And then as quick as that, she sashayed away. But the seed had been planted, the 'damage' was done. I had seen that look in the eyes of many a fellow dinner or party guest before . . . this was not my first rodeo.

'I'm on a diet, you know. The <insert favourite diet>. I have been on it for <insert time frame> long. I wanted to do it because of <insert illness or reason>. I did a lot of research before I started, and I have lost <insert amount of weight lost>, and feel so much better. What do you think?'

And then the whole rest of the evening is spent on this very topic.

It wasn't my wife's first rodeo either, and the moment Karen dropped the 'D-word', Jane sashayed away with Karen, mumbling about finding another drink or something else to eat . . . Cowards!

In truth, after a couple of glasses of Malbec, I'm game to talk about most things.

'Guess how old I am?'

(I didn't want to . . . *please don't make me*)

'Fifty-eight. I know I don't look it . . .'

(He did look it.)

'About a year ago, I starting getting a little worried about my health and thought I needed to tone up and lose a bit of weight.'

Then followed a long litany of his research into various diets that I won't bore you with, during which another glass of Malbec and more canapés were consumed.

'Anyway, what I ended up sticking with is the Carnivore Diet. I've been on it for nearly a year now.'

Pardon me now? I couldn't help myself, so I asked:

'Carnivore Diet? That is where you largely eat meat?'

'Oh no, I eat ONLY meat . . . and eggs and a bit of dairy.'

Ooookayyy . . . 'Umm, and what about vitamin C and fibre?'

'Even though you are supposed to be fine, I take a multivitamin just in case. And nope, not one bit of fibre! The only side effect is my poop [I have substituted poop for the actual word he used; this is a family audience after all] is really smelly and like pellets . . .'

I have a very sharing face. People often share all kinds of stuff with me, and sharing, after all, is caring . . . but I think you'll agree that this had now entered the realm of too much information.

'I mean, maybe I'll drop dead tomorrow of a heart attack! But it's been nearly a year and I feel great! I've lost a ton of weight and I am ripping it in the gym . . . here, feel my arms . . .'

I didn't want to feel his arms, but he put my hand on his biceps anyway.

Yes, this is the kind of thing that happens at parties when I'm drunk enough to let on what I do or, in this situation, when somebody else let's on what I do!

The Carnivore Diet is the most extreme of the 'low-carb, high-fat' family of diets that include Keto and Atkins. And, if you hadn't noticed, the Carnivore Diet is also very high in protein. So does

Carnivore work? It seems to have benefitted John, and apparently hasn't killed him (yet). But if it does work, then how?

I BLAME MY HORMONES

In essence, calorie for calorie, meals higher in protein appear to be more filling. The question, of course, is why?

In order to appreciate how high-protein diets work, we first have to understand why and when we feel hungry or full. When we feel hungry, all of us get a grumbly stomach. Dinner – beef short-ribs braised in a rendang (a Malaysian coconut curry) sauce – is currently in the oven as I am writing this passage and as I smell the fragrance throughout the house, my stomach is getting chattier and chattier. Sometimes it can get really quite loud as well, so much so that others within our immediate vicinity can hear its apparent cries. Incidentally, these sounds emanating from a grumbly stomach are a consequence of the peristalsis in the stomach and small intestines moving gastric juices and gases about. It actually happens pretty much all of the time, but when there is food in the space, it muffles the sound. Thus the rumbling is quite literally the echoey sound of an empty stomach. As a consequence, it is natural for most people to consider the feeding centre to be at the level of the stomach. However, while the stomach undoubtedly does play a role, we now know that it is the brain that controls all of our feeding behaviour.

Our brain needs to know two key pieces of information in order to control food intake. First, it needs to know how much fat we are carrying. Why? Because how much fat we are carrying, which is our long-term energy store, is a marker for how long we would survive in the wild without any food. Not a common problem today, clearly, when we have too much food. But you have to remember that for the vast majority of human existence we didn't have enough food. So knowing how long our energy stores would last is a useful integer to hold in your head. This piece of information is relayed to the brain by hormones secreted from fat into the bloodstream where they are then sensed by the brain.

The second piece of information your brain needs to know is how much and what you are currently eating, or have just eaten. These are short-term signals that are going to come from your food-to-poop tube, your gastrointestinal tract. When we take a mouthful of food, from the moment we begin chewing till the moment it emerges from the other end, hormones are secreted at every step of the way. As food makes its way through our gastrointestinal tract, hormones are released in response not only to how many calories are in the meal, but crucially, its 'macronutrient content' as well – that is, how much protein, fat and carbohydrates are present. Let's take my beef short-rib rendang for dinner tonight, which I am serving with steamed rainbow chard, carrots and peas, together with plain white rice. What if I asked you to take a stab at how many calories are in the meal, and its macronutrient content? I could certainly try to come up with an educated approximation . . . but who am I kidding, any numbers I came up with would just be a guess! Here's the thing, though: as the meal travels through our gastrointestinal tract and is processed and digested, the repertoire of hormones that are released informs our brain of exactly how much fat (probably a bit too much because short-ribs are a fatty cut, which is what makes them sooo unctuous and delicious), protein and carbs it contains. Our brain senses and integrates these long-term and short-term hormone signals and then influences our next interaction with a supermarket, kitchen fridge or restaurant menu.

Gut hormones

Hormones are any signals that are released from one organ and transported by blood to target another distant organ in order to regulate physiology or behaviour. Insulin, for example, is a hormone released by the pancreas and transported by the blood to a number of target tissues, signalling to our muscles, for instance, to take up glucose. Hormones are therefore our body's long-distance 'command and control' system. An 'endocrine' organ is any that produces hormones, and by that definition our gut is actually the largest endocrine organ in the body. The hormones released by our gut play a crucial role in regulating how hungry or full we feel, particularly in the period immediately after a meal.

Our gut, especially the small intestine, is lined with delicate single layer of cells called the gut epithelium. These cells are 'polarised', meaning they are directional, with one end sticking into the gut lumen and the other in contact with blood vessels. The luminal end of a gut cell has tiny finger-like protrusions known as villi in order to maximize the surface area to absorb nutrients, and the close contact of the other end with blood vessels allows the absorbed nutrients to be transported to where they need to go quickly and efficiently. This single layer of cells has to tread a fine line, making sure that vital nutrients are allowed through while keeping bacteria, potential toxins, and anything else destined for the poop-end of the tube, out of the blood supply. Thus, these cells work very hard and are replaced every few days, but they do not produce any hormones.

However, about one in every hundred cells of the gut epithelia do a very different job. They are known as entero-'endocrine' cells, and their role is not to absorb nutrients, but rather to sense them as they travel through the gut and to release hormones into the blood in response. There are at least fifteen different types of enteroendocrine cells and they are characterised both by the types of hormones they release and where they are localised within the gut. Some of the types of cells are localised in the stomach or in the duodenum, right at the top of the small intestine, some are localised lower down in the ileum or jejunum and down into the large intestine, while others are found along the entire length of the gut. They also appear to be named by someone who was eating a bowl of alphabet soup with their children at the time; called, as they are, D cells, G cells, I cells, K cells, L cells, S cells, etc. OK, to be fair, many of them were named after the primary hormone they secrete (or are thought to secrete). For example, G cells in the stomach secrete gastrin that stimulates gastric-acid secretion, and S cells in the duodenum and jejunum produce secretin, which stimulates secretion of digestive enzymes from the pancreas. Others, however, such as the L cells, secrete GLP-1, oxyntomodulin and PYY ... Maybe the 'L' in GLP-1? Anyway, together, these gut entero-endocrine cells are responsible for releasing around twenty different hormones that play such a critical role in regulating our appetite. I go through only a few of them in this chapter. If you want to find out more, take a look at this review from my colleagues at Imperial College in London.[1]

What is interesting is that the vast majority of these gut hormones, when they signal to the brain, make us feel full. CCK or cholecystokinin, for example, is released from I cells in the duodenum and is very short-acting, with its 'feel-full' effect lasting less than thirty minutes, thus it is likely to play a role in signalling when you should stop eating. In contrast, PYY or peptide YY, which is secreted by L cells primarily in the ileum and large intestine, has effects that last many hours, bridging the gap between meals, and therefore influencing how much you are likely to eat from one meal to the next. One of the exceptions to the 'gut hormones make you eat less' rule is ghrelin, which is produced by the stomach and makes us feel hungry. In fact, ghrelin levels in the blood rise acutely just before a meal, triggering hunger and playing a role in when we choose to eat.

Your brain doesn't sense and respond to each of these hormones in isolation. Rather, as different foods – each with their own unique ratios of fat, protein and carbs – are consumed and digested, the mix of nutrients are sensed by the different enteroendocrine cells as they travel down the gut. This results in the release of a complex repertoire of gut hormones, from which, somehow, our brain is able to accurately determine the nutritional and caloric content of the meal. Is it not just a bit annoying, though, that our brain doesn't feel the need to let us in on the secret?

Except, it sorta does, just not in way that we can easily enunciate. Anecdotally, we all know we feel different, better or worse, more or less full, after we have eaten different meals. But it is more than anecdote, because multiple studies over the years have shown that depending on the macronutrient content of a meal, we will feel more or less full. Meals higher in protein, for instance, appear to be more satisfying. Put simply, a calorie of protein makes you feel fuller than a calorie of fat, than a calorie of carb, in that order.

Why does protein make you feel different to fat or carbs?

WEIGHT-LOSS SURGERY AND A SERENDIPITOUS DISCOVERY

While we have known about the satiating effect of protein for some time, our understanding of why this was the case came later, with serendipity, as so often is the case, lending a helpful hand. It came about as a result of scientists trying to develop surgical methods to tackle the rapidly increasing problem of severe obesity, so called bariatric (from *baros*, which is Greek for weight) or weight-loss surgery. As the doctors began to get their heads around this new type of surgery, it completely changed our appreciation of the way gut hormones functioned, and ultimately how our gut works.

There are a number of flavours of bariatric surgery available; some that are more effective than others, and some that are more permanent than others. And as it turns out, the less permanent approaches are also the least effective. An example of this is the gastric band. A gastric band is a silicone ring that is placed around the stomach near its upper end, close to the oesophagus. This creates a small pouch with a narrow passage into the remainder of the stomach below the band. For a patient this means that after eating a small amount of food the small upper pouch becomes full, thereby making the patient feel full. The gastric band also has an inflatable balloon on its inner surface that is connected to a small device placed under the skin (usually near the middle of the chest). This is so the band can be tightened or loosened after surgery, which then decreases or increases, respectively, the rate at which food can move out of the small pouch, allowing a doctor to adjust the amount of food the patient can eat before feeling full. It isn't a severe intervention, relatively speaking, and because the band can be removed, neither is it permanent. The approach works as it is designed to, by limiting the amount of food that can enter the stomach. While effective, the gastric band doesn't result in as much weight loss as other methods, and critically if the band is removed, the food restriction stops and the weight comes back on.

The most frequently used of the permanent bariatric surgery methods is one called Roux-en-Y gastric bypass or RYGB. It is incredibly effective, not only leading to around ten kilograms of weight loss over a period of four weeks after surgery, but also a reversal in the type 2 diabetes seen in many people living with obesity. Crucially, the weight loss is maintained years after the surgery. In this procedure, the upper section of the stomach is first stapled off, leaving a small pouch of about thirty millilitres in volume, so just a couple of tablespoons; then this new smaller stomach is attached directly to a part of the small intestine lower down, the jejunum. This means that the majority of the stomach and the attached initial section of upper small intestine, so the entire duodenum (which is about 0.4 metres) and about 0.6 metres of the jejunum, has literally been clipped out and bypassed (hence the name), shortening the food-to-poop tube by a metre and change. The surgery has, in effect, 'replumbed' the gut. The section of bypassed gut, however, is not removed; rather, it is reconnected to the new main flow of the small intestine, just below where the now smaller boutique stomach meets the small intestine. Why not just remove the leftover stomach and one metre of gut? Why leave it flapping around inside our body? This is because, if you recall from Chapter 3, a number of accessory organs secrete enzymes and other substances directly into the duodenum as part of the digestion process. The pancreas, together with Brunner's glands within the duodenum wall, secrete bicarbonate to neutralise the stomach acids; the gall bladder secretes bile, which emulsifies fat; and a whole suite of pancreatic digestive enzymes, including lipases, amylases and trypsins are released to begin the process of chemical digestion. All of these enzymes are still released into the duodenum, which is now a cul-de-sac that no food can get to, and without them, digestion can't occur. So by connecting the duodenum to where the 'new' stomach meets the jejunum, the enzymes empty into where the food now enters the small intestine, and digestion can proceed.

When RYGB was first conceived, it was designed to function in part like the gastric band – by reducing the size of the stomach, hence making you feel full with less food – and in part by reducing the amount of nutrients that are absorbed, owing to the shortening of the small intestine. There probably is a minor effect of reduced absorption, and a short-term impact of the ridiculously small stomach making you feel full faster. However, because the stomach is very flexible, it begins to stretch quite rapidly and before long, the same volume of food can fit into the stomach again. So amazingly (or depressingly, depending on your point of view) the stomach very rapidly adapts and is not a significant limiting factor on the amount of food that is able to be consumed post-bypass. Why does the gastric band work where the removal of the majority of the stomach doesn't? I don't think we know entirely, but the fact that there is the adjustable band acting as a synthetic barrier, thus preventing the stomach from adapting, as opposed to simply the removal of most of the stomach, probably plays a role.

So if it isn't the smaller stomach size or reduced absorption, how does RYGB work to achieve and, importantly, to maintain weight loss? Two key observations of patients pre- and post-RYGB have transformed our understanding not only of how the procedure leads to weight loss, but also of how the gut works. First, many people (although not all) with obesity also suffer from type 2 diabetes, and this is therefore also true for the people with severe obesity that end up getting bariatric surgery. What doctors observed was that after RYGB, the patients' diabetes improved dramatically; in many cases, patients could actually reduce or even stop their anti-diabetic medication. But this, in of itself, was not a shock, because if carrying too much fat led these folk to get diabetes, then surely losing weight would then reduce the risk of diabetes. It was the speed at which this occurred that really surprised doctors, with improvements in diabetes happening less than twenty-four hours after the surgery, clearly before any notable weight loss could have occurred![2] Second, after the surgery, many patients reported a sudden change in eating behaviour, once again beginning before any notable weight loss.[3] Not only did they feel full faster, but their taste in food also changed. Many found a sudden love of salads and found fatty foods to be less appealing, for instance. Hmmmm . . . an overnight change in feeding behaviour? Curiouser and curiouser.

There are two potential explanations for such rapid systemic and behavioural change. The 'replumbing' that has occurred could have led to changes in direct communication from the gut, via the nervous system, to the brain. It is certainly plausible that this plays some role. However, the most straightforward explanation for such rapid change is changes in hormonal secretion. Hormones, after all, are designed to respond dynamically to internal and external challenges, and to affect rapid changes to physiology and behaviour. When scientists measured some of the gut hormones pre- and post-RYGB, they found a number of them to be raised post-surgery. There was, for example, a large rise in GLP-1, oxyntomodulin and PYY post-RYGB, all of which are produced from the L cells. While L cells are found in small number in the duodenum and jejunum, they are primarily found lower down in the ileum and in the large intestine.

The further down the small intestine food travels, the more chemical digestion that occurs and the more nutrients that are absorbed. These are then sensed by the alphabet soup of entero-endocrine cells that are interspersed down the length of the gut, which secrete hormones in response. In RYGB, because a metre of the upper small intestine has been bypassed, food arrives lower down the gut in a less-digested state than it would normally be. This different nutritional mix is sensed by the enteroendocrine cells, which then change the amount of hormones they secrete in response. This change in hormonal levels is what mediates many of the changes seen post-RYGB.[4]

GLP-1, for example, is known as an 'incretin'; it promotes the secretion of insulin by the pancreas. If you infused someone with glucose directly into their veins, insulin levels would go up. If, however, you ate the glucose as part of a meal (say as starch or as sucrose), it would obviously have to go through the gastrointestinal tract and get absorbed in the gut. Because of the involvement of the gut, in addition to a rise in insulin levels, GLP-1 levels also go up, which then signals to the pancreas. The involvement of GLP-1 amplifies insulin secretion by 50 to 70 per cent, thereby improving the ability of our muscles and fat to take up glucose from the blood. This is the so-called 'incretin' effect and has led to GLP-1 analogues being used as an effective treatment for type 2 diabetes. Thus, the increase in GLP-1 secretion post-RYGB will have played a role, together with other hormones, in the rapid reversal of type 2 diabetes in patients.

And what about the dramatic and sustained weight loss? As we now know, most gut hormones make us feel full. Thus, the rise in blood levels of a whole host of gut hormones post RGYB, including that of GLP-1, oxyntomodulin and PYY, is sensed by the brain, making the patient feel fuller and, in many patients, even appearing to change their feeding behaviour. What happens if you feel fuller? You will, naturally, end up eating less. In fact, patients who have undergone RYGB eat a lot less, explaining the dramatic weight loss, and they carry on eating less for years and years after, thereby explaining the sustained weight loss.

So, while RYGB did not function at all like it was designed to, it nonetheless turned out to be an incredibly effective intervention. RYGB, in fact, is currently (at time of writing) the only known long-term 'cure' for obesity and, for many, type 2 diabetes as well. I put the word 'cure' in inverted commas because it is debatable whether reversing obesity and/or type 2 diabetes is truly a cure in the way that someone is cured from a broken leg, the flu, or a kidney stone, for instance. Might a better term be 'in remission'? Meaning that either obesity or type 2 diabetes could return with a change in environment? Anyway, I'll return to this discussion later in the book. Crucially, the efforts to understand how RYGB actually worked in turn revealed new biology about how the hormones in our gut interact with our brain.

So, wait, what does this have to do with high-protein diets again?

Patience, young padawan. It all comes together in the next couple of sections.

WEAPONISING OUR GUT HORMONES

OK, so what if RYGB is an effective intervention? For some folk it is not hyperbole to say the treatment is life changing, lifesaving even. However, I am certainly not countenancing rolling out

RYGB to the entire population. It is, after all, a major surgery with associated mortality, even if it can now be performed laparoscopically (by keyhole surgery), and also, if I can remind everyone, it is permanent.

What happens, however, if you can mimic the post-gastric bypass hormonal mix without the actual surgery? Could we perhaps 'weaponise' our gut hormones, and 'trick' the brain into thinking it is full? Scientists at the Imperial College, Hammersmith Hospital in London, led by professors Tricia Tan and Sir Steve Bloom, are doing exactly this experiment. They began, more than a decade ago, by infusing patients with the hormones GLP-1, oxyntomodulin and PYY individually, and showing that each hormone on its own could modestly reduce food intake. Over the years, they have systematically tried different doses and combinations, and are now at the stage of trialling an infusion of all three hormones in a single mixture.[5] While the treatment is still in the testing phase, it appears that this hormone infusion can indeed mimic gastric bypass, at least partially, and make the brain think it is full so patients actually eat less, around 30 per cent less in a single meal! There are hurdles to clear, of course, the biggest of which is how to make the infusion more long lasting. At the moment, you have to inject the hormones before every meal. The goal is to be able to inject these hormones once a week and get the same effect. The holy grail in fact is to get these hormones into pill form, but because of the pesky acidic cauldron that is the stomach, that is a long way off yet. Nevertheless, these results are very exciting indeed and represent really significant progress in obesity therapeutics.

PROTEIN MAKES YOU FEEL MORE FULL

However, for the majority of people, the most important and relevant way of weaponising our gut hormones does not involve either replumbing our innards or big needles before each meal, which will undoubtedly come as good news to many. One of the key lessons learnt from bariatric surgery is that if food that is less digested than it should be is delivered, because of the bypass, further along down the gut it triggers the release of a hormone mix that signals to the brain to make you feel full (or fuller). What if we considered that lesson from a different perspective? What would happen if, rather than shortening the gut, one were to simply eat something that takes longer to digest? As it turns out, because food that takes longer to digest would then end up travelling further down the gut, it has the similar effect of making you feel fuller.

I mentioned earlier that a calorie of protein makes you feel fuller than a calorie of fat, than a calorie of carb, in that order. Another way to look at it would be to say that meals that have a higher protein content are more satiating. These are two related but distinct concepts really: feeling full, which is a spectrum that can go from gently pleasant to deeply unpleasant; and being satiated, which means to be satisfied, and is most certainly a positive feeling. A major reason that protein makes you feel fuller is simply that it takes longer to digest than fat and carbs. How about why protein is more satiating? Well, that is a more complicated question and has to do with the range of signals it induces. A big part of the answer is because it triggers the secretion of gut hormones that make you feel fuller, as I've mentioned, but it is more than that. Eating more protein increases the concentrations of amino acids in the blood, as well as that of the various fragments (known as metabolites) of amino acids that form during their metabolism. A higher-protein diet is also often coupled with a reduction in carbohydrate consumption, which can result in an increase in ketone production. All of these signals are sensed by the brain and play a role in satiety. Then there is the issue of the thermogenic effect attributed to the metabolism of protein, which is far more than that for fat or carbs. Protein synthesis, the high ATP cost of peptide-bond synthesis and the high cost of urea production all result in increased energy expenditure in the form of heat. This increase in thermogenesis is also thought to play a role in the satiating effects of protein.

As a result, and this may or may not come as a surprise to some of you, there is actually plenty of evidence to support the effectiveness of diets 'high' in protein for weight loss, at least in the short-term.

Now, what does 'high' mean, exactly? As it turns out, that is a surprisingly difficult question to provide with a straight answer. The amount of protein in our diet can be considered in different ways: as an absolute amount of protein in grams; the amount of protein ingested per kilogram of body weight; or the percentage of total energy (calories) ingested as protein. Using this last measure, the WHO (World Health Organisation) recommends that the amount of protein we eat should account for around 10 to 15 per cent of the total number of calories consumed a day, as long as you are in energy balance and weight stable, i.e. not trying to gain or lose weight.[6] Where there is data available, the numbers from different countries indicate that what is being consumed reflects these recommendations. Protein intake in both the UK and the US, for instance, is a little higher, at around 16 per cent of total daily calories for a sedentary adult. This equates to about 64 grams per day for the average female and 88 grams per day for a male.

I know what you are thinking (because I thought it too), that 88 grams sounds like a miniscule amount! But remember that 88 grams refers to pure protein. For example, I love steak, in particular the king of cuts, the ribeye. In a typical restaurant, the serving size for a ribeye steak is about 300 grams (raw weight). There are of course many places that serve far larger portions, and a number of high-end fancy-shmancy places that will serve you a far smaller portion. Many people think that steak is pure protein with a bit of fat. Not true. So 100 grams of ribeye actually contains around

19 grams of protein and 15 grams of fat, which equates (using the Atwater factors of 4 calories per gram of protein and 9 calories per gram of fat) to 211 calories. But 19 grams + 15 grams is only 34 grams. What about the rest of the steak? Well, most of the weight of the steak, the remaining 66 grams, is composed almost entirely of water! That would mean that chewing your way through a full 300-gram ribeye would still only get you 57 grams of protein. What if you decided to splash out on the leanest and most expensive of cuts, the fillet (or loin, or filet mignon, depending on where you call home)? A hundred grams of raw beef fillet contains 23 grams of protein and 5.5 grams of fat, which is 141 calories. Although there is more protein per gram of fillet compared to a ribeye, fillet steaks are typically served in 200-gram portions, which would be 46 grams of protein. As it turns out, most lean meat, such as chicken or fish, also has around 20 per cent protein. Of course, protein is not only found in meat. An egg would have 6 grams of protein each, and protein accounts for 25 per cent of most nuts and dried lentils; although we don't eat dried lentils, of course, and cooked lentils contain 9 grams of protein per 100 grams. My point is that 88 grams is actually quite a bit of protein, equivalent to a 450-gram ribeye, fourteen and a half eggs or nearly a kilogram of lentils. And it is important to note, for all you vegetarians and vegans out there, it is the amount of protein rather than their source that is crucial to satiety[7], which means that a range of protein sources can contribute to satiety, including dairy, meat, poultry, cereals, fish, peas, pulses and legumes.

The issue is that there is no general consensus as to what constitutes a 'high'-protein diet. The food industry does use the term 'protein enriched' for anything that contains 20 per cent protein from calories, but that is used to describe individual food items. So because there is no definition of what a high-protein diet is, most research papers that assess its effectiveness tend to include all diets that have more than 16 per cent of the calories from protein. And effective it apparently is. For example, in a review paper that summarised the main findings of fourteen studies comparing 'high' protein to at least one other macronutrient, eleven found that high protein significantly increased subjective ratings of satiety.[8] The perennial issue with dietary studies is that when using actual foods it is difficult, if not impossible, to conduct a proper 'randomised control trial'; the gold standard for assessing the effectiveness of a particular intervention. When you are testing whether a drug works, you can have a control pill with white powder, and participants in the clinical trial are then 'randomised' to the control or the drug. Crucially, the participant doesn't know if they are in the control or the experimental group, so there is no bias. You clearly can't do this when using actual food, because there will be differences in flavour, texture and calories. So one just needs to realise this when attempting to interpret comparisons between different diets.

The bottom line is that because protein is less calorically available than fat or carbs, our bodies have to work harder to extract the calories from protein. For all of the reasons discussed above, this then drives its satiating effects, and explains how the vast majority of dietary approaches that involve the element of increased protein intake work.

#LCHF DIETS

The interesting thing is that most of the recent popular diets (a rapidly moving feast, pun intended) that look, smell and act like high-protein diets barely mention protein in their publicity bumf, at least not in the headline section. Rather, most focus their wrath and ire on the evils of carbohydrates, and many extol the benefits of fat. These fall under the broad church of 'low-carb, high-fat' diets, and if you happen to be *au fait* with the world of social media, it even has its own hashtag, #LCHF, used to flag up posts on Insta-gram (#IG, #insta, #thegram) or Twitter and proudly adorning the biographies of avid practitioners. As an aside, I'm mystified by why one would feel the need to broadcast whatever dietary approach they happen to be following. Perhaps declaring it publicly is akin to signing a contract, so they now have no choice but to go through with whatever dietary restriction is involved? Actually, I get that. Is there an innate need to be identified as part of a group or com-munity? Hmmm . . . am I beginning to answer my own question? Perhaps misery, indeed, loves company (OK, OK, don't @ me, that was said in jest . . . sorta). Anyway, not judging, just musing.

You might think that #LCHF would be a modern phenomenon, and certainly the hashtag is of the moment, however, the low-carb concept is much older. Surely then it must have begun with Rich-ard Atkins and the eponymous diet he founded when he published his book *Dr Atkins' Diet Revolution* in 1972[9] (and another sixteen books after that, until he died in 2003)? Most of us would probably consider the Atkins Diet the father of the fad diets, or it is, at least, the first diet most of us would have ever heard of, and the one most of us could still name today. Without the Atkins Diet blazing the blockbuster fad-diet trail, the diet industry of today would, in all probability, be a very different beast.

But yet, there was actually a 'low carber' that preceded Atkins by more than a hundred years.

William Banting was born in England in 1796. He was an un-dertaker and, at least earlier in his life, was obese. He was five foot five inches and at his heaviest was 202 pounds; this would have been very large indeed for someone in the 1800s. Banting clearly didn't like being obese and made multiple unsuccessful attempts at trying to lose weight, until he happened upon a dietary change that finally worked for him. In 1863, now a svelte 167 pounds, and as one is wont to do, he wrote a book describing his diet plan – well, book might be too strong a word as it was succinct at eighteen pages. The booklet (a better term) was called *Letter on Corpulence, Addressed to the Public*, and, in the best tradition of diet books, even in the nineteenth century, was written in the form of a personal testimonial.[10] 'Corpulence.' I mean, is there a more Dickensian word to describe one's body size?

Banting wrote:

'. . . *my corpulence and subsequent obesity was not through neglect of necessary bodily activity, nor from excessive eating, drinking, or self-indulgence of any kind . . .*'

Umm, if it wasn't excessive eating or drinking or indulgence, what could it be? Then in the same sentence:

'. . . *except that I partook of the simple aliments of bread, milk, butter, beer, sugar and potatoes more freely than my aged nature required . . .*'

Facepalm. OK, so it clearly was due to excessive eating and drinking!

Banting then consulted with a close doctor friend who recommended (and I include the quote for you to enjoy the lovely use of language):

'. . . *increased bodily exertion before my ordinary daily labours began, and thought rowing an excellent plan. I had command of a good, heavy, safe boat, lived near the river, and adopted it for a couple of hours in the early morning. It is true I gained muscular vigour, but with it a prodigious appetite, which I was compelled to indulge, and consequently increased in weight . . .*'

Please raise your hands if you feel his pain? No judging! Let those who have never felt compelled to indulge a prodigious post-bodily-exertion-induced appetite cast the first stone. That's the problem with using exercise as a weight-loss strategy; exercising makes you feel hungry! 'You can't outrun a bad diet' is the typical refrain. Except you can, if you are Mo Farah or Paula Radcliffe or any other elite endurance athlete who consumes thousands upon thousands of calories a day when training; it's just that most of us mere mortals don't run or swim or cycle for long enough to burn off the calories we feel we need to eat after exercise. However, while not a particularly good tool for weight loss, there is good evidence that it is effective for weight maintenance. I also feel compelled to add that even if you don't lose a single gram in weight, nothing can replace the positive benefits of being physically active.

Banting then goes on to describe his failed attempts at fasts, diets and various spa regimens until at last, upon some advice from yet another friend, he happened on a successful formula. Banting wrote that there were certain foods that one could eat without limitation when young – one might even go so far as to describe them as beneficial – but which then became prejudicial in later life.

'*The items from which I was advised to abstain as much as possible were: Bread, butter, milk, sugar, beer, and potatoes ... These, said my excellent adviser, contain starch and saccharine matter, tending to create fat, and should be avoided altogether.*'

Banting gave up these foods that contained starch and saccharine matter (carbs, in effect), and lost 35 pounds in thirty-five weeks. In 1863, Banting became the first 'low-carb' influencer. His pamphlet was popular for years to come and has become a foundational text for the modern low-carb movement.

Even today, the so called Noakes Diet, championed by controversial and evangelical #LCHF advocate Dr Tim Noakes,[11] is often referred to as the Banting Diet in his native South Africa.

LOW-CARB MENU

After William Banting's 'low-starch and low-saccharine-matter' diet came the phenomenon that was Lulu Hunt Peters in the early 1900s – whom we met in Chapter 2. Peters was an advocate of calorie counting, though, and strongly disapproved of cutting out individual food groups. So the next low carber to come along and take up Banting's mantle was indeed Richard Atkins, more than a century later, in 1972.

At its inception, the Atkins Diet was focused almost entirely on counting carbs, with no headline mention of high fat. However, in common with the emporium of different diets in the #LCHF movement that followed, the stated aim of Atkins was to transform the body's metabolism from one that stored fat into one that burnt fat. The argument went something like this: high-carbohydrate diets raise blood sugar, which in turn signals the pancreas to secrete more insulin, higher insulin levels encourage fat storage and a sugar-burning (as opposed to a fat-burning) metabolism. So, reduce carbs, reduce insulin, burn more fat and lose weight! Yay! The Atkins diet plan (there has to be a plan otherwise it's just not credible) is a four-step process: induction, which gives your weight loss a jumpstart; ongoing weight loss, which gets you down to your target weight; pre-maintenance, which tries to prevent any immediate rebound; and maintenance, which is the long-term strategy to keep the weight off.[12] Each step in the process differs in the amount of carbs you are allowed to have.

All of the #LCHF diets (try to) differentiate themselves from one another on their websites and associated promotional bumf by touting differing philosophies, and I am using the word 'philosophies' here with all the baggage that it comes with. But they all follow the same broad principle, with cosmetic variations to the plan, differences in types of food allowed and, crucially, the severity of carbohydrate restriction.

The Dukan Diet, for example, follows a very similar four-step plan. In fact at first glance it seems almost identical to Atkins. The big difference is that the Dukan Diet highly restricts the type of foods that you can eat. According to their website:

'*The Dukan Diet will redesign your eating habits and help you permanently stabilise your weight. The Dukan Diet is a high-protein, low-fat, low-carb diet – a healthy eating plan based on proteins and vegetables, 100 foods in total. And what's best, it's EAT AS MUCH AS YOU LIKE.*[13]

It really is quite a restrictive diet . . . with only one hundred foods you can eat, but without limit! Could you really live the rest of your life eating only one hundred different types of food? Perhaps the real trick to losing weight is by becoming bored to death with your food.

There is also the summery, surf-shorts and bikinis South Beach Diet,[14] which is another variant of Atkins. The difference being that in the South Beach Diet there isn't only a restriction in the amount of carbs that one can eat, but also the type of carbs. It ranks carbohydrates according to their 'glycaemic index', the amount by which they will raise blood glucose levels (we'll look at glycaemic index or GI in detail in the next chapter), and only allows consumption of those on the lower end of the GI scale – so-called 'healthy' carbs.

#KETO

Then moving towards the more extreme end of carbohydrate restriction is the Ketogenic Diet, often contracted to Keto (or #keto on all of the socials). Keto is a type of #LCHF, but most #LCHF do not count as Keto. That's because most #LCHF diets, including Atkins, Dukan and South Beach, contain too much carbohydrate! Keto is a high-fat, moderate-protein, very-low-carbohydrate diet. There is so little carbohydrate in the diet that there ends up being little to no glycogen stores in the muscles and liver, which forces much of the body to burn primarily fat. The combination of increased fat oxidation and very low dietary carbohydrates results in a slowdown of the Krebs cycle and a glut of acetyl-CoA (which, if you recall, I describe in eye-watering detail in Chapters 3 and 4). When this happens, the liver, through a process called ketogenesis (hence the name of the diet) converts the excess acetyl-CoA into ketones. These ketones are then transported by the blood, and all cells with mitochondria (with the exception of liver cells that make ketones but can't use them) can then take up these ketones, which are then converted back into acetyl-CoA and used as fuel. The rate of ATP production is initially slower when relying on ketones, but our body is able to metabolically adapt over time.

Ketogenic diets have actually been around for a long time. They have been used in a clinical setting since the original version was designed in 1921 by Dr Russell Wilder at the Mayo Clinic in Rochester, Minnesota, to treat particularly hard to control epilepsy in children.[15] The exact mechanism has still not been fully unravelled, but forcing the brain to use ketones as fuel rather than its favoured glucose seems to reduce the number of seizures that occur. In 2013, Keto began creeping beyond the epilepsy field when a group in San Francisco published research demonstrating that one of the ketone bodies with the chemical name of β-hydroxybutyrate could activate antioxidant and anti-inflammatory genes.[16] This was, at the time, interpreted by the press to mean that the Keto Diet could slow the ageing process . . . ![17] Over-egging the pudding slightly. Anyway, by 2015, Keto had entered the weight-loss vernacular, and by 2017 it was 'the new black', the zeitgeist in diets.

The classic Ketogenic Diet, which was originally used for the management of seizures, had 80 to 90 per cent of calories come from fat, 5 to 15 per cent come from protein, and 5 to 10 per cent come from carbohydrates. While keto is sold as a high-fat, ultra-low-carb diet, the reality is that most people cannot manage the more than 80 per cent fat that is recommended. It is an extreme level of fat that is quite unpalatable to many. You wouldn't, for example, eat a stick of butter (ick . . . or maybe you could, I'm not judging): butter on toast, however, fat and carbs, mmmmm. As a result, a modified version called the 'standard Ketogenic Diet', which allows you to eat more protein (from 20 to 30 per cent of your total calories) but with the same carbohydrate restriction is the version of the diet most commonly used today. Thus, the diet, as it is currently deployed, is very high in protein, as compared to the 15 per cent protein in today's typical western diet.

IT WORKS, JIM, BUT NOT AS WE KNOW IT . . .

Here's the thing, there is actually pretty good evidence that these #LCHF diets, all of which increase the protein-to-carb ratio to varying degrees, work for weight loss, at least in the short-term. The all-important questions are why and how?

What of the claims that these diets restrict foods that are known to raise blood sugar and insulin, and that limiting carbohydrates forces your body to use fat for energy rather than sugar? Well, the first of these assertions is, actually, broadly correct. Carbohydrates, in whatever form they are consumed, cross the gut wall and enter the blood as glucose. So carbs will indeed raise blood glucose faster than either fat or protein. Because insulin secretion from the pancreas is very sensitive to blood glucose levels (as long as one does not have type 1 diabetes), then insulin levels are sharply raised by carbohydrates.

The second assertion is only partially correct. Limiting the amount of carbohydrates consumed will also limit the amount of glycogen stores, which does mean your body turns to using fat more quickly. But there are organs and cells in the body that either don't or cannot burn fat. The brain, for instance, doesn't use fatty acids as fuel, and relies primarily on glucose – although it can, if required, obtain up to 50 per cent of its energy requirements from ketones. Also, because red blood cells don't have mitochondria they cannot use fatty acids and have to rely on glucose. As a result, blood glucose levels, as long as one is not diabetic, are tightly regulated, even while on a ketogenic diet, to make sure your brain and blood cells are fuelled. Of existential importance, I think you would agree. So while we can be low-carb in our diet, our liver will continue to pump out glucose that it has converted from the breakdown products of fat and protein through gluconeogenesis. Whether we use carbs or fat as fuel also depends very much on what exactly it is we are doing. So at rest, our body primarily will use fat to power our basal metabolic rate. During short bursts of activity, however, the preferred fuel of our muscles, because of the speed it can be deployed, is glucose. As we transition over to more than a few minutes of activity and longer endurance events, our muscles then shift back to oxidising fat. Although if you recall from my escapade cycling up a mountainside in France, when I burnt through all of my glycogen stores and ended up 'hitting the wall' the presence of a little bit of dietary glucose actually makes the burning of fat far more efficient. We have evolved to be able to use ketones as an important energy substrate under certain conditions, most importantly during starvation, and they can indeed modulate carbohydrate and lipid metabolism. A ketogenic diet functions by mimicking certain metabolic aspects of starvation. However, under normal physiological conditions, our body prefers to utilise a blend of fuels in response to the situation at hand.

WHERE ARE THE CARBONS COMING FROM?

How about the key #LCHF argument that higher insulin levels encourage fat storage? Reducing carbs means reducing insulin, means burning more fat, and that is why #LCHF results in weight loss ... Once again, there is a kernel of truth to this assertion. When insulin levels are raised, this does indeed push your body into storing fat. However, insulin triggers the storage of all nutrients, from the building of muscle from protein, to the generation of glycogen from carbs, not just fat-storage.

The absolutely critical thing to remember is that if you eat too much of anything – fat, protein or of course carbs, aside for a *soupçon* of glycogen (about 2000 calories' worth) – the spare nutrients will be turned into and stored as fat; the average person carries around 110,000 to 180,000 calories of fat, depending on sex and size. So the key question to ask is where is the energy coming from? Or, from a metabolic perspective, where are the carbons coming from? Even if insulin levels do rise sharply, as they do after a carb-rich meal, it can only promote storage of energy that has been consumed and is there in the body. Equally, when insulin levels drop, triggering the breakdown of energy stores, the drop in fat mass sensed by your brain will drive you to eat more. The only way to gain weight is to eat more than you burn, and the only way to lose weight is to burn more than you eat. It is a fundamental law of physics, and there is no way of getting around it. Antoine Lavoisier, Max Rubner, Wilbur Atwater and Lulu Hunt Peters all knew this.

So why do high-protein diets work for weight loss? Because of the simple fact that protein is less calorically available and therefore more satiating, for all the reasons we have discussed in this chapter. In addition, if you push yourself into ketosis, there is evidence that ketone bodies also signal to the brain and contribute to the feeling of being less hungry. If you are less hungry and more satiated, you are going to eat less; if you eat less, you will achieve a calorie deficit; if you are in calorie deficit for long enough, you are going to lose weight. That is pretty much the whole nine yards.

GLUTEN-FREE

There are other diets with hugely complicated backstories and explanations for how they might work, but they also come circling back to the satiating effects of protein. Going 'gluten-free' is one.

A common misconception is that gluten is a type of carbohydrate, which it isn't. It is actually a composite of proteins found in a number of grass-related grains such as wheat, barley, rye, oats and their various related species. Gluten (from Latin *gluten* or 'glue') is 'activated' when flour meets water, and the resulting dough is kneaded. This activated gluten provides the characteristic elasticity of dough, allowing it to capture the carbon dioxide produced by yeast metabolising sugar to form millions of air bubbles, thus making bread rise.

About 1 per cent of humans have coeliac disease, which is an autoimmune condition triggered by the ingestion of gluten that attacks and eventually destroys the delicate single-cell layer of the gut wall. Given that the cells in the gut wall play a central role in digestion, nutrient absorption and hormonal signalling, coeliac disease is a very serious condition indeed. For people suffering from the disease, the only 'cure' is to give up gluten for life. Then there are folks with 'non-coeliac gluten sensitivity', a term used to describe individuals who have a negative coeliac diagnosis, but have symptoms, ranging from mild to severe, related to ingestion of grains that contain gluten. The number of people with gluten sensitivity is less certain because of the spectrum of the severity and the difficulties to diagnose at scale, but it is thought to be around 3 to 4 per cent of the global population. So that is about 5 per cent of humans with some form of gluten intolerance. Yet 25 per cent of us buy explicitly labelled gluten-free products because we think they are somehow healthier, even if there is no scientific evidence to suggest that this is actually the case. Gluten-free has become such a selling point that manufacturers are now labelling things gluten-free that never contained gluten in the first place. Gluten-free rice, gluten-free corn, even gluten-free water. Most ridiculous of all are that inedible products are being marketed as gluten-free as well. Gluten-free shampoo! I mean, come on!

So why is gluten thought to be bad? In essence, the argument is that since gluten can cause problems in a small percentage of the population it must be wreaking havoc on everyone's gut lining, turning our intestines into sieves. I have written about the byzantine 'science' that conclusively demonstrates the evils of gluten in far greater detail in my previous book, *Gene Eating*.[18] Gluten, as a result, has been blamed for everything from type 2 diabetes, obesity, heart disease, cancers, all manner of autoimmune conditions, and Alzheimer's disease, just to name a few. And the testimonials about the benefits of going gluten-free are many and glowing, with the diet embraced by the Hollywood glitterati, Instagram gurus and elite athletes alike.

The reason why it is so very popular is because it works for many people. Weight falls off, six-packs and chiselled jaws magically appear, type 2 diabetes goes into remission, and skin begins to 'glow'. What does that even mean? Does our epidermal layer begin to auto-fluoresce?

So why does going on a gluten-free diet work, particularly for weight loss? In North America and Europe, because wheat and rye are such a ubiquitous source of carbohydrates, a gluten-free diet essentially means a pretty restrictive low-carb diet. This also means a corresponding increase in calories from fat and protein. Thus a gluten-free diet is, in effect, #LCHF, which is how it works for weight loss.

But what about all of the other magical effects of giving up gluten?

Because obesity is a risk factor for so many other diseases including type 2 diabetes, heart disease, certain cancers, and also neurological disorders such as Alzheimer's, losing a large amount of weight reverses type 2 diabetes in most (but not all) people and reduces the risk for all the other diseases.

PALEO

Another popular diet, this one with a backstory more epic in timescale, is the Paleo Diet. The term 'Paleo' is a contraction of Paleolithic, which is a prehistoric period going from about 2.6 million years back to the dawn of agriculture about 12,000 years ago. The diet was so named because it was designed to mimic the diet of indigenous populations prior to the agricultural revolution. The basic premise for the whole Paleo movement was that for the vast majority of human existence, since *Homo sapiens* emerged 200,000 to 300,000 years ago, we subsisted as hunter-gatherers. Then the dawn of the agricultural revolution some 12,000 years ago brought about huge changes to our diet. Since diet-related illnesses are responsible for much of the chronic and non-communicable disease burden today, and no evidence of such conditions can be seen in the Paleolithic skeletal record, the blame for our contemporary woes must lie with the post-agricultural diet. Hence, the solution must surely be to shift back to a pre-agricultural, so-called 'ancestral', subsistence.

Many books and websites are available that detail the intricacies of the Paleo lifestyle or diet.[19] However, there are pretty much only two basic sets of ground rules that you need to follow: a) what you SHOULD eat is lean meat and seafood, as well as fruit and non-starchy vegetables, which can be consumed without limitation, because these would have been available in the Paleolithic; b) what you SHOULD NOT eat are cereals and grains, starchy root vegetables, legumes, dairy products, alcohol and processed foods, because these are the fruit of agriculture.

There are a number of problems with this argument. First of all, there was no single Paleolithic diet, because there was no singular Paleolithic people. There were humans hunting and gathering on the African savannah, on the arctic tundra and in the Amazonian rain forests. Rather, hunter-gatherers ate what was available to them at the time, depending on their environment; they were adaptable. Second, the reality is that we are not eating what our ancestors ate, because we can't. Those foods simply no longer exist. Almost everything that we eat today is a product of many generations of domestication. So the complex backstory is really quite nonsensical, and the notion that anything we are eating today is similar to some supposed ancient diet is simply fantastical.

But yet, there are still many avid disciples of the diet. Why? Because humans love a great story (which it is) and, more importantly, it does actually work as a strategy for weight-loss, at least for some. Additionally, there are claims, very much like the ones made about going gluten-free, that 'going Paleo' is a panacea for diseases such as type 2 diabetes and insulin resistance, multiple sclerosis, rheumatoid arthritis, coeliac disease, cancer, heart disease, osteoporosis and anaemia.

Why and how does this diet work? Just go back to those simple rules again; eat lean meat and seafood, as well as fruit and non-starchy vegetables, and avoid cereals and grains, and starchy root vegetables. It is, once again, #LCHF, though not by name, which is why it is effective for weight loss. 'That which we call a rose by any other name would smell as sweet,' said some dude once. As for the reduction of all the other diseases? It is the same domino effect we see when people go on a gluten-free diet. A significant drop in weight would be enough to reduce the risks for all of the diseases for which obesity is a risk factor.

CARNIVORE

Finally, we come full circle back to my Christmas soirée and that gentleman who had been on the Carnivore Diet for nearly a year.

The Carnivore Diet is a restrictive diet that only includes meat, fish, and other animal foods like eggs and certain dairy products.[20] Although carnivorous aficionados also recommend eliminating or limiting dairy intake to foods that are low in lactose, such as butter and hard cheeses. It excludes all other foods, including fruits, vegetables, legumes, grains, nuts and seeds.

The Carnivore Diet is on the extreme end of the #LCHF diet, because it pretty much excludes all carbs. It is also at the extreme end of the Paleo Diet. The Carnivore Diet actually stemmed from the belief that our Paleolithic ancestors ate mostly meat and fish and little to no carbs. But as I touched on above, this comes from the 'Fred Flintstone and his brontosaurus ribs' school of pre-history; i.e. fantastical. It is true that if you were an Inuit in the Arctic your diet might have been rich in seal and whale meat and blubber. However, if you were on the African Savannah or the Serengeti, you would have, in all likelihood, been largely vegetarian, given how difficult it would have been to actually track, let alone take down, an antelope.

In the short-term, considering the extreme restrictiveness of the diet, you can see how it would work very effectively for weight loss. Protein, satiation, caloric deficit, blah blah blah. However, with no fruit or vegetables and no fibre, how healthy can it be, even in the medium term? I am surprised that the dude at the Christmas party had lasted, if you take what he said at face value, nearly a year on the diet! And given his smelly pellet-like poop (sorry to bring up the image again), I'd be willing to bet that his gastrointestinal tract and the bacterial denizens within would have been screaming for mercy. No one has yet conducted any studies into the safety of the Carnivore Diet for any length of time, but I'm going to stick my neck out here, and call this particular fad diet a bad idea.

IS #LCHF HEALTHY?

So can we eat too much protein? Almost certainly, given that too much of anything will end up being bad for you. I guess a better question to ask is whether an #LCHF approach is sustainable for health in the long-term.

Well, as you might expect, 'it depends'. We can consider the answer in three parts.

First, high protein. When most of us consider high protein, we immediately think of meat. But the satiating effects of protein are apparent, whatever the source of the protein, whether animal or plant based. Too much meat, particular that of the red and pro-cessed variety, has been shown to increase your risk of certain cancers, such as colon cancer. The consensus from the literature indicates that a moderate intake (200g per day) of white meat, such as chicken and turkey, shows no increased risk, whereas consumption of fish appears to have a beneficial effect. The American Cancer Society (ACS), Cancer Research UK, the British Heart Foundation and the UK NHS advise minimising the intake of processed meats such as bacon, sausage, lunch meats and hot dogs, encourage us to choose fish, poultry, or beans instead of red meat (beef, pork and lamb), and if eating red meat, to choose lean cuts and eat smaller portions.

Thus, if you are omnivorous, a balance of animal-based and plant-based protein will undoubtedly be the best course of action in the long-term.

How about if you are vegetarian or vegan? Because different foods have different amino-acid compositions, and amino-acid mix is tricky to measure, and changes depending on how the food is prepared, the best practice is to eat a mix of protein. Don't only eat chickpeas or tofu as your sole source of protein. 'Eating the rainbow', or keeping a range of colours of food on your menu, is as useful a strategy to use for pulses and nuts as it is for leafy vegetables. Variety is, after all, the spice of life, and that is certainly very true for sourcing your protein.

Second, low carb. We can certainly survive easily without consuming sugar in its powdered form, and it is probably wise to stay away from too many refined carbs, such as white flour. There is even some evidence that a low-carb diet, keeping carbs at 20 per cent of total energy intake, could help mitigate the inevitable regain in weight that occurs when a person loses weight.[21] It would, however, be difficult to eliminate carbohydrates entirely from your diet. For one thing, cutting out carbs completely makes it difficult to get enough fibre, which is critical for long-term health (see next chapter). Yes, you can get fibre from fruit and vegetables with very few carbs, but it remains the case that fibre from whole grain continues to be an important source. Additionally, healthy sources of carbohydrates, such as higher-fibre starchy foods, vegetables, fruit and legumes, are also an important source of nutrients, such as calcium, iron and B vitamins. Significantly reducing carbohydrates from your diet in the long-term could mean you do not get enough nutrients, potentially leading to health problems.

Finally, high fat. This is going to entirely depend on your source fats. If you are replacing carbohydrates with animal-based protein and fats, then the likelihood is you would increase your intake of saturated fat, which can raise the amount of cholesterol in your blood. Cholesterol gets a bad rap because high levels in the blood are associated with increased risk of heart disease. In fact, it is all too easy to forget that this molecule is critical to our survival. Cholesterol is an essential component of cells, giving cell membranes their structure, that all-important mix of rigidity and flexibility. Without cholesterol, we would, essentially, be a puddle on the floor. It is also an important component for the manufacture of bile acids, steroid hormones, as well as several fat-soluble vitamins. Cholesterol is insoluble so it has to be moved about in the blood by fat-transport proteins called 'lipoproteins', which come in different flavours, including low-density lipoprotein (LDL) and high-density lipoprotein (HDL). LDL carries cholesterol *to* the cells that need it. High levels of LDL cholesterol, however, are associated with heart disease, which is why it has acquired the moniker of 'bad cholesterol'. That's because when levels are high, LDL cholesterol is taken up by immune macrophages, which are engorged to form foam cells that become trapped and accumulate in the walls of blood vessels, forming plaques. This contributes to atherosclerosis, or a stiffening and narrowing of the blood vessels, leading to serious problems, including heart attack, stroke, or even death. In contrast, 'good' HDL moves cholesterol *away* from cells, removing and transporting it from the circulation back to the liver for excretion. Eating unsaturated fats in place of saturated fats has been shown to reduce 'bad' LDL cholesterol, thus improving your cholesterol profile. These are going to come from either fish or plant-based sources. Crucially, for some people, their cholesterol levels, because of their genetics, are not actually influenced by their diet at all. They can add or remove whatever they want from their diet, and their cholesterol levels are not going to budge.

So is #LCHF safe in the long-term? The answer is, it all depends on your sources of protein and fat, and the severity of the carbohydrate restriction. If you are getting your protein from a mix of plant- and animal-based sources (or colourful plant-based sources if you are vegan), eating more unsaturated than saturated fats, and lowering your carbohydrate consumption in a moderate fashion, then this version of #LCHF is healthy, safe and sustainable in the long-term. At the other end of the spectrum, we have Keto. As I mentioned, while the Ketogenic Diet works in the short-term for weight loss, there were, at time of writing, no published studies into its long-term safety. Given its popularity, these are important studies that need to be carried out urgently.

As for Carnivore, I cannot see, from first principles, how it can be safe given its extreme restrictiveness; in particular its complete lack of fibre and high animal-based protein and saturated-fat content. Perhaps I will be proven wrong, and someone will one day show that we humans can somehow remodel our whole omnivorous physiology to that of a tiger.

Actually, no, I won't.

I think it is safe to say that it will never be a good idea, for our health or for the planet, for humans to eat meat and only meat.

CHAPTER 6

The wonder of fibre

'My internet connection and my diet are missing one thing in common . . . Fibre'

Dad joke on the internet

I am, and always have been, an honest-to-god 'meatatarian'. I eat all manner of vertebrate species, roasted, BBQ'd, burgered, cured, tartared . . . you name it, I love it. So when the producers of the BBC's *Trust Me, I'm A Doctor*, on which I am one of the presenters, asked me to go on a vegan diet for a month, it gave me pause for thought. Actually, in truth, just the thought of it terrified me! But glancing down at my mid-forties and slightly wobbly belly, and knowing that my cholesterol levels were a tad high, I recognised an opportunity to be grasped, and grasped it.

Veganism as a diet is easy enough to understand. You just have to avoid consuming anything animal based, including dairy and eggs. In contrast, the reasons motivating people to become vegan are complex. To some, it is a philosophy deeply rooted in ethics, while others are driven by the environmental impact of the meat industry. Many, however, choose a vegan diet to become healthier, which was the angle the producers tasked me with investigating.

Whatever the reasons people choose to become vegan, it is undoubtedly one of the (if not *the*) fastest-growing food trends. At the beginning of 2019, Beyoncé and JAY-Z, the American power couple of R&B and hip-hop, even offered the chance for fans to win lifetime (!!) tickets to their shows, as long as they were incorporating plant-based foods (more on this later) into their diets! If I needed any added motivation to give this a good old-fashioned go, then this was it!

Before leaping in with both feet, I spent quite a bit of time researching and planning (with military precision) how exactly I was going to implement a vegan diet. First of all, I went through all of the food in my kitchen to identify the items that were clearly meat- or dairy-based, which was, for the most part, a straightforward task. Closer reading of the back of packaging, however, revealed quite a few surprises. While most dried pasta is vegan, some has egg in it; there are powdered soup-bases for some instant ramen noodles which, while suitable for vegetarians, actually contain milk protein; and who knew oyster sauce actually had bits of oyster in it? OK, maybe I should have known about the oyster sauce.

Now with my eyes zeroed in on the minute levels of pesky non-vegan ingredients in foods that were otherwise entirely vegan, I began to loiter around supermarket aisles to try and find out just how 'healthy' vegan food actually was. Clearly it would not be controversial to consider whole fruits and vegetables as healthy. The issue becomes mired in complexity when foods are 'processed', a loaded term if there ever was one. The word 'processed' encompasses a broad church; curing, drying and pickling are processes, so is the simple act of applying heat to a food – cooking or pasteurisation, for example – and all of these techniques have allowed us humans to extend the shelf-life of food and reduce the chance of being poisoned. So the processing of food has increased our chances of surviving, which is clearly a good thing. What about the contemporary industrial processes that have given us the vast midsections of our favourite supermarkets that are set aside for confectioneries to suit all tastes? These processes have further extended the shelf-life of food, sometimes indefinitely, making transport and storage far easier, and, importantly, driving down their cost. These are critical characteristics of contemporary food that allow the planet to sustain its seven billion (and rising) human inhabitants. However, while calories today in most developed economies are plentiful and cheap, these 'ultra-processed' foods, which I will consider in detail in the next chapter, are typically stripped of much of their nutrients and fibre, and contain higher levels of sugar, fat and/or salt in order to improve flavour.

What I realised was that a large percentage of these ultra-processed foods are certified to be vegan, hence vegan food, per se, was not necessarily 'healthy'. I could have, for instance, spent the entire month eating crisps, cookies and any number of other vegan confectionery items, of which there are many. I even found a 'bacon-flavoured' snack that claimed to have no artificial flavouring, yet was certified to be vegan (go figure). As an aside, I did figure it out. When I saw the packet, I read 'no artificial *bacon* flavouring', whereas these 'bacon' rashers were clearly naturally flavoured, with smoked paprika or turmeric or some other proxy of bacon flavour, say.

VEGAN VS PLANT-BASED

Then there is the difference between being vegan and being 'plant-based'. First, there are differences in the reasons why people choose to identify as one over another. Most people choose to be vegans for ethical reasons or environmental reasons or both. Folks who practice plant-based living, however, do so because they believe that animal-based protein will be harmful to their health, and their health is their primary motivation for eating this way.

A plant-based diet is also more strict than a vegan diet. Food is considered vegan so long as it does not contain animal parts or derivatives. So a plant-based meal is in effect 'food from plants', and would clearly be suitable for vegans. However, while all plant-based food is vegan, the reverse is not true. There are all manner of ultra-processed foods that are free of animal products, but are not suitable for people sticking to a whole-foods, plant-based diet (by whole food I mean minimally processed food). Examples include liquid calories such as soda, energy drinks, and other sweetened beverages; refined foods such as those made with bleached flour and refined sugars; and foods containing chemical additives such as artificial colourings, flavourings, and preservatives, including dairy-free pastries and low-calorie soda. Tofu and its by-product soy milk are plant-based; and so is coconut milk.

For my month-long experiment, I elected to stick to a whole-foods, plant-based diet. Why? First of all, I didn't want to be that guy who went vegan for a month and gained weight, on camera to boot, that would have been seriously crap! Second, and more importantly, this was a health programme after all and I wanted to see how healthy being vegan could be. A plant-based diet, as op-posed to heaps of chips, crisps and faux-bacon rashers, certainly seemed to me a better bet for my waistline.

On the day I was to start, I travelled up to Coventry University to visit with dietician Dr Duane Mellor. He poked and prodded me and gave me a 'once over' in order to establish some base-line values of health (or not!). I was weighed and had taken some lim-ited blood biochemistry measurements (glucose and cholesterol levels, and micronutrients), and then I was let loose on the vegan world.

As I arrived at Nuneaton train station (the closest station to Coventry) to head back south to Cambridge, I paused in front of the coffee shop and stared longingly at the array of baked goods on display. There would be thirty long days before I could enjoy these muffins and pastries, all steeped in butter and eggs, again. So I took a good long sniff of the glorious aroma, triggering a suspicious glance from the lady behind the counter, and walked away.

FIRST WEEK EPIPHANY

Although I had read many vegan cookbooks and reached out to 'cheffy' friends for advice about how to obtain 'umami' flavour without using meat (I can now do magic with miso), the first week did not go so smoothly. There was a disastrously sloppy quinoa concoction, although the blame there falls squarely on the cook (me) and not the quinoa. There was also an unhappy liaison with some oat-milk 'crème fraîche'. Before anyone yells at me, it didn't taste bad, it just didn't taste like crème fraîche. The manufacturers managed to achieve the initial citrusy flavour profile of crème fraîche (from oats!), but it faded away in two nanoseconds to end up tasting like white emulsion paint (OK, it did taste bad . . . to me at least).

And that was when I had my epiphany. When I prepared a dish that was meant to have dairy or meat, and replaced it with something else, then I missed the meat. For example, I made a 'cottage pie' but swapped out the minced beef for lentils. While I did manage to make it taste nice, it simply did not taste like beef . . . but why would it? Whereas if I made something that was never designed to contain meat to begin with, then there was nothing to miss, and life became easier. So what did I eat? For one thing, I ate a lot of tofu, which, being Chinese, I was raised on. It could be firm tofu, used more in stir-fries, silken tofu, used in soups, or fried 'puff tofu', which can be used for anything – curries, stir-fries, soup, even on the BBQ! In and of itself, tofu has a neutral flavour, not tasting of anything much. It does, however, act like a sponge, soaking up the flavour of whatever sauce it is cooked in. Typically, if tofu was used in a dish, it was as the primary protein element, so there was no meat to miss. Dishes that were well spiced also worked for me; my famous five-bean chilli and a whole host of vegetarian Indian curries and dahls, for example.

But then, tofu, beans and lentils are protein rich.

One thing that did surprise me was the ease with which you could be vegan outside the controlled environment of the house, at least within the UK. This was true not only in the fancier eating establishments, but in most pubs and regular restaurants as well, where there were almost always multiple vegan options on offer, all clearly marked. It was even true for my local Indian takeaway, where they cheerfully replaced ghee with olive oil, allowing me to continue to indulge in my regular Friday-night curry. Life would (possibly) not have been worth living otherwise!

I did have an interesting experience at a restaurant in Cambridge, which I found very informative about the broader dietary trends today. I was out for dinner with some friends, all of who were feeling sorry for me, incidentally, and told the waiter that I was vegan, just to make sure there were no inadvertent animal products in the food (yes, I had become 'that guy'). After he helpfully pointed out the vegan options to me, he then asked, 'Are you gluten-free as well?'

I was slightly taken aback, if only because there was no biological reason for someone on a vegan diet to avoid gluten, unless they were coeliac or gluten-intolerant. Clearly, however, enough people were coming into the restaurant that were vegan and avoiding gluten, or gluten-free and avoiding animal-based products (yes, there is a philosophical difference!), for the waiter to have asked. It appeared that someone on one dietary restriction, at least in Cambridge, was also more likely to be on some other restriction. Given that there is no ethical or environmental reason to avoid gluten, that particular restriction would have almost certainly been for some mythical health reasons.

THE PICTURE OF PLANT-BASED HEALTH?

Before I knew it, twenty-nine days had passed (not that I was counting), and I was heading back north to Coventry for my end-of-diet poking and prodding by Duane.

One thing that I did not need Duane to inform me was that I had lost weight. I, like most people, have a set of bathroom scales, and I had been tracking my weight daily during my diet, so I knew my weight had been falling away. My trousers were looser and I had to pull in my belt to the last available notch. It was visible as well, with my normally very round cheeks becoming just a little less round. In fact, when I got to the University of Coventry and was met by Mike Duffy, one of the *Trust Me* producers, he greeted me by saying, 'Wow, Giles, you're looking gamey!'

I had lost 4 kilograms or 10 pounds in weight over the month, pretty much at an even rate. And I was, to be honest, thrilled! Additionally, I had no vitamin or mineral deficiencies as a result of the diet, including the all-important vitamin B12. Crucially, for my longer-term outlook, my blood cholesterol levels dropped by 12 per cent, from 6.4 millimoles down to 5.6 millimoles!

Would you take a look at that; weight loss, no vitamin deficiencies and better cholesterol numbers! On the face of it, I appeared to be the poster boy for vegan living, the picture of plant-based health! But here is where the (vegan) meatballs meet the sauce. Why did I apparently become 'healthier'? Was it specifically because of the plant-based diet, per se?

WHAT IS FIBRE?

One unequivocal characteristic of plant-based diets is that they are incredibly rich in fibre, which, together with protein, is the other critical component that influences the caloric availability of food.

So what is fibre? Well, dietary fibre is actually a plant-derived carbohydrate; it is the part of plant-based food that humans cannot digest. Fibre can be divided into two components, soluble and insoluble fibre, both of which are found in all plants in differing proportions.

Soluble fibre is so called because, as reflected in its name, it dissolves in water. In fact, some types of soluble fibre actually attract water, turning into a gel. Pectin, the natural gelling agent in soft fruit that allows you to turn them into jam, and gelatine, which is used to make jelly or panna cotta, are both soluble fibres. When this happens in the gut, this gel of dissolved soluble fibre actually slows down digestion, which, as we discovered with protein in Chapter 5, has the effect of making you feel fuller for longer. Once it gets down to the large intestine, it is also fermentable by the resident bacteria of the gut, producing goodies such as short-chain fatty acids, as well as making you feel gassy – more about this on page 179. Soluble fibre is found in oat bran, barley, nuts, seeds, beans, lentils, peas, and some fruits and vegetables.

Insoluble fibre is just that, insoluble. It is what most people think about when the word 'fibre' is mentioned; the skin of fruit and root vegetables, and the fibres in vegetable stems and leaves. It is completely inert to any of the digestive enzymes, juices and bacteria that are found in the gut. So it goes right through you and out the other side. What it does is add bulk to your poop, speeding up large intestinal transit, thus helping you be regular in your *ahem* bowel movements. It is found in foods such as wheat bran, vegetables, and whole grains.

There is a third class of carbohydrates that are resistant to digestion, but are not technically considered a fibre (although they are often spoken of in the same breath), and these are 'resistant starches'. Starch, as you know, are chains of glucose, and are eminently digestible, beginning with salivary amylases, all the way through to the small intestine. Resistant starches are, however, because of their structural configuration, resistant to digestion in the small intestine, but are then fermented by the gut bacteria in the large intestine. Resistant starches are found naturally in certain foods, like unripe bananas, for instance. As bananas ripen, the resistant starch they contain gets converted to normal digestible starch. They are also formed by the cooling and reheating of certain carbohydrate-rich foods, including pasta and rice.

How did fibre go from being something that took a lot of chewing and that you pooped out, to become this apparent panacea for health?

BURKITT'S FIBRE HYPOTHESIS

The credit for crystallising and then disseminating the link between the consumption of fibre and health goes to the British surgeon Denis Burkitt – so much so that it actually bears the name 'Burkitt's fibre hypothesis'.[1]

Denis Burkitt spent twenty years of his career, after the Second World War, working in Uganda, where he was interested in the geographical patterns of diseases such as cancer. In 1963, Burkitt became renowned in medical circles when he described the distribution and cause of a specific childhood cancer of the jaw that was subsequently named after him: Burkitt's lymphoma.[2] I mean, how often is something named after you, let alone two things? But he clearly had an eye for detail and patterns. While Burkitt was working in rural Uganda, he noticed that middle-aged folks there (forty to sixty years old; OMG, I'm middle-aged . . .) had far lower incidences of diseases that blighted people of similar age living in England, including colon cancer, diverticulitis, hernias, varicose veins, diabetes, atherosclerosis, and asthma. These so-called 'Western diseases' are all associated with lifestyles commonly led in high-income countries. The other thing that Burkitt noted was the typical diet of the locals, which was low in red meat and animal fat but high in starch and fibre-rich foods, such as colourful fruits and vegetables, leafy greens, tubers, potatoes, beans, nuts and whole grains. This high-fibre diet (50 to 120 grams per day) resulted in bulky stools, which speedily transited through the colon, and was associated with a relative absence of 'Western diseases', including colon cancer. In comparison, the fibre content of the average British diet in the 1960s was around 15 grams per day, similar to what it is today.

Burkitt left Africa and returned to England in 1966, largely because of changes that were occurring in post-independence Uganda. His plan was to continue his research into the geographical distribution and incidence of cancer in Africa, with support from the UK's Medical Research Council (MRC), who, incidentally, also fund my research on obesity today. The plan was certainly not to implement a wholesale shift in his programme of research and to begin looking into fibre. While the fibre hypothesis is named after Burkitt, he did not come up with it in an intellectual vacuum. There was also unlikely to have been a single eureka moment for the fibre hypothesis; rather, as is the case with many great ideas, it was a result of a synthesis of evidence from different sources.

Between 1966 and 1972, there were a number of people who influenced Burkitt's thinking. For instance, Dr Neil Painter, an expert in diverticulitis – a condition where small pouches, called diverticula, form in the lining of the large bowel and push out through the gut wall, causing unpleasant symptoms – was convinced that fibre, or lack thereof, played a key role. He gave patients suffering from the condition bran, which is high in fibre, and their symptoms improved.[3] Then there was Dr Alec Walker, a Scotsman who emigrated to South Africa and started a lifetime of research into disorders he thought were related to diet, poor nutrition and prosperity. He studied the role of fibre in heart disease, and also showed that bowel transit was much slower in white South Africans than in black South Africans, who, as a population, had a higher-fibre diet and rarely suffered from bowel cancer.[4] Dr George Campbell, and in particularly Dr Peter Cleave, were also both interested in the causes on 'Western disease'; Campbell on type 2 diabetes in particular, whereas Cleave was interested in all of what he called 'modern' diseases. However, neither ever invoked the importance of fibre, but rather focused on what was left behind once the fibre had been removed. Both blamed the consumption of sugar and re-fined carbohydrates as the common factor. Cleave went so far as to write an influential book on the subject, encapsulating these ideas, and naming this cluster of modern diseases 'saccharine diseases'.[5]

It is interesting, therefore, that Cleave was the person who argu-ably most influenced Burkitt's thinking. On the occasion of their very first meeting, having been introduced by a mutual friend, Burkitt actually remarked in a personal diary entry, 'Time and chance happen to all men'. No other record of that conversation was kept, but it was quite clear from Burkitt's subsequent writings that he was never sold on the sugar story.[6] One crucial message that Burkitt did take from Cleave was the idea that if diseases clustered together, both in their geographical distribution and in the same patients, then they were, more likely than not, to have a common or related cause.

In discussion with all of these people and many others, Burkitt put the pieces of the fibre story together and was finally respon-sible for telling the world about it. In 1969, he published in the medical journal *The Lancet* his hypothesis:

'Benign and malignant lesions of the large bowel which show such a relationship are examined, and it is suggested that there is epidemiological and other evidence to incriminate low-residue diet as a major aetiological factor.'[7]

By 'low-residue' diet, Burkitt meant a low-fibre diet, with refer-ence to the residue that is left over after digestion and absorption has occurred. While this first iteration of Burkitt's Fibre Hypothesis related specifically to bowel cancer, it soon extended to include all of the other, to employ Cleave's parlance, 'Saccharine Diseases'.[8]

FIBRE AND HEALTH

Over half a century later, fibre intake in Western high-income countries still struggles to come anywhere close to the more than 50 grams per day advocated by Burkitt. For example, in the US today, the average fibre intake is about 16 grams per day and in the UK, not much better at 18 grams per day. This is against a background of rapidly increasing incidence of type 2 diabetes and obesity. Obesity wasn't even a significant public health issue in the 1970s, only becoming a measurable problem in the US in the mid-1980s, yet today, the worldwide prevalence of obesity and all of its myriad co-morbidities – including diabetes, heart disease and certain cancers – are rising rapidly, particularly in middle-income and low-income countries around the world, with numerous studies confirming the association between low-fibre and high-glycaemic index diets with type 2 diabetes and obesity in particular.[9]

We now know, from multiple epidemiological studies, that significantly increasing the fibre content of our diet either decreases the risk of, and in some cases protects against, a number of different non-communicable diseases. For example, a study based on data from the European Prospective Investigation into Cancer and Nutrition Study (EPIC), which involves 519,978 participants from ten different European countries, showed a 40 per cent reduction in cancer risk when low-intake populations doubled their fibre intake.[10] In support of the overarching Fibre Hypothesis, a large systematic review of fifty-eight clinical trials encompassing 4635 individuals suggested a 15 to 30 per cent decrease in all-cause, cardiovascular-related stroke, type 2 diabetes and colon-cancer mortality (deadness), as well as a decrease in incidence of all these diseases, when comparing the highest dietary fibre consumers with the lowest.[11] Crucially, more is better in this case, with fibre intakes higher than 35 grams per day appearing to be even more effective at reducing disease risk. Thus there is substantial evidence that a diet high in fibre might not only reduce colon cancer risk and deaths, but also all cancer deaths, and all-cause mortality, possibly even increasing lifespan.

So why is dietary fibre so very good for us? Three reasons. First, it is critical for good bowel health. In many ways, this is a purely mechanical explanation and includes making sure that bowel muscles stay strong, and that everything is emptied regularly. Your faeces, after all, are waste products, and while our gut is designed to store this waste for a period of time, you don't want this (literal) 'crap' hanging about in your body for longer that it needs to. Also, the longer faeces stay in the large bowel, the more water is removed, the harder it gets and the more difficult it becomes to evacuate. This leads to constipation, where the whole food-to-poop tube is plugged up. As you might imagine, this situation is deeply unpleasant and would not be tenable for any length of time, so it is important to keep your whole system moving and on some form of schedule!

The other two reasons are a little less visceral but of no less importance to our health. One has to do with the interaction between our gut bacteria and the fibre that we consume, and the other with reducing the caloric availability of the food that we eat.

HOW DO OTHER ANIMALS HANDLE FIBRE?

While our gastrointestinal tracts are unable, largely, to extract the energy tied up in fibre, there are many other mammals, ruminants in particular, whose digestive systems are adapted to do just that.

What is interesting is that they have had to enlist 'external' help in order to do so.

There are around two hundred different species of ruminants, including, for example, cows, sheep, goats, deer, giraffes and camels. 'Ruminant' comes from the Latin *ruminare* meaning 'to chew over again', reflecting a digestive system that is very different from our own. Ruminants are all herbivores, and instead of one chamber to the stomach, they have four. The first and largest of the compartments is the eponymous rumen, which together with the second smaller compartment, the reticulum, contain billions upon billions of symbiotic microorganisms that have been 'externally' co-opted (although they obviously live and are cultivated internally) to help in the digestion process. These are largely bacteria, although they also include some yeast and fungi, and their role is to break down the cellulose and other insoluble fibre found in grass, leaves and other robust vegetation. In effect the rumen and reticulum act as a microbiological fermentation vat. Ruminants, like cows, first partially chew their grass–buttercup–dandelion salad and this munched-up concoction then enters the rumen to be fermented. The rumen is really quite a voluminous chamber; a cow's rumen is around 120 to 200 litres in size, for example, which allows for a great deal of grass–buttercup–dandelion salad to be consumed and then fermented into balls of 'cud'. Once sufficiently fermented, the cud moves to the reticulum, which is made of muscle, and by contracting, forces the cud into the cow's oesophagus and back up into the mouth. There it goes through a second round of mastication, before it is re-swallowed (mmm mmm ... delicious). This process of swallowing, un-swallowing, re-chewing and re-swallowing is called 'rumination', or more commonly 'chewing the cud'. After being re-swallowed, the twice-chewed and fermented cud then enters the third compartment, the omasum, which sort of acts like a giant filter to keep larger chunks of plant particles inside the rumen, while allowing fluid to pass through. This just gives the bacteria in the rumen more time to break the chunks down; the more broken down, the more available the calories. After the plant fragments are broken down to a small enough size, they eventually pass through the omasum and into the 'true stomach', the abomasum. It is, as with our stomachs, an acidic cauldron of gastric acids and juices, where chemical digestion (as opposed to microbiological fermentation) begins, and the broken-down vegetation goes from there into the small intestine for the bulk of the digestion and nutrient absorption to occur.

The digestive system of ruminants enables them to utilise the energy tied up in the cellulose and fibre found in grass and other plants that animals with one stomach, such as humans, dogs and pigs, cannot digest. Over 50 per cent of the energy in grain and cereal food crops is inedible to humans. Thus ruminants have the ability to convert these plants and residues into high-quality protein in the form of meat and milk, which we can then consume.

THE BUGS IN OUR GUT LOVE FIBRE

While we uni-stomach humans don't have the luxury of possessing a rumen, we do, as with most creatures possessing a digestive tract, have an entire ecosystem of microorganisms that live within us; our microbiome. There is a famous (scientific) urban myth that there are more bacterial denizens in our gut than we have cells in our body. This, as it turns out, is apocryphal; there are probably the same number of bacteria in us as we have cells . . . which still number in the trillions and that is still an awful lot of zeroes! The gut microbiome has evolved through a symbiotic relationship with the host (us), to perform a multitude of tasks; in particular shaping our immune systems to provide protection against pathogens, helping to maintain our intestinal barrier integrity and influencing our metabolism and our ability to absorb nutrients. Over the past decade or more, our bacterial symbionts have been linked to the development of, or protection against, a whole array of different diseases, including obesity, diabetes, heart disease, autoimmune conditions, dementia, schizophrenia and other mental-health conditions. In fact, the microbiome has been linked to such a broad range of conditions, almost every disease it seems, that it has led to an inevitable backlash, with a large section of the scientific community vocally expressing their scepticism of the field, describing it as over-hyped.

So is studying the microbiome good science or bad science? Personally I think it is still a new science. What we definitively know about our gut bacteria is that it is a wonderful reflection of our health (or unhealth . . . is that a word?) and the environment we are living in, and the part of the environment that most directly influences the microbiome, is of course our diet. How about what makes our microbiome healthy or unhealthy? The problem is that too many people try to answer this question too definitively, saying bug X and Y are most certainly good for us, whereas bug Z we need to get rid of. Whereas the appropriate mixture of bacteria in each of us is likely to depend, in part, on our genes, with one of the big challenges being to understand the interaction between the microbiome and our individual immune systems. The other big challenge is trying to determine if our gut bacteria go beyond simply reflecting disease to actually driving or causing disease, or can it even be used to cure disease? Say we have a skinny person and a person with obesity – will there be a difference in repertoire of bugs that live in each person? In all likelihood, yes, reflecting the possible differences in diet and health. Can you, however, take the bugs purified from the poop of the skinny person, transfer them over to the heavier person, and make the heavier person lose weight (or even vice versa, but that would be ethically questionable)? This process is known as faecal microbiota transplantation – also called a 'transpoosion' if administered via the back end, so to speak, and if the bugs are encapsulated in a capsule to be swallowed (don't think too hard about it) it is called a 'crapsule', and, no, I'm not making any of this up. While data from mouse experiments looked hopeful, the few human trials that have been conducted have shown the transplantation to have no effect on bodyweight.[12] So from these initial, admittedly small, studies, it seems unlikely that the bugs are playing a major role in driving or causing obesity. Further high-quality human studies will be required to provide more definitive answers about the microbiome's link to other diseases.

What is clear is that we need a healthy and varied microbiome, not only to keep our gut in tip-top shape, but also for our overall health. How might the microbiome be contributing to our health? While our gut bacteria are different from those found in ruminants and are unable to break down insoluble fibre, they do play an important role in fermenting soluble fibre within the large intestine, and as a result releasing so-called short-chain fatty acids, or SCFAs, as metabolites. Depending on the substrate that is being fermented and broken down, a number of different SCFAs – primarily acetate, propionate and butyrate – are produced. Increasing evidence now implicates these SCFAs as key mediators of the beneficial effects of the gut microbiome.[13]

Acetate tends to cross the wall of the large intestine and enter the bloodstream. It can be used as fuel by the muscles, can regulate the release of fatty acids by fat cells and can also signal to the brain to help regulate appetite. Propionate acts locally in the gut by binding to receptors on enteroendocrine L cells to stimulate release of the gut hormones PYY and GLP-1. A small proportion of propionate gets into the blood and ends up in the liver, where it can either be oxidised or used in gluconeogenesis to produce glucose. Butyrate's actions are largely confined to the gut, where it plays a key role in helping maintain the gut barrier, allowing water and nutrients through, while keeping bacteria and everything else destined for the poop shoot out. All three SCFAs also play a role in regulating blood pressure.

Given that SCFAs sound like some kind of panacea for health – even possibly reducing appetite and food intake – why are we not advised to sprinkle them on our cornflakes or toast in the morning? So here's the thing: eating SCFAs does not appear to have any effect in humans, at least on food intake, either during a test meal or over the twenty-four-hour period following consumption. SCFAs that are consumed orally have to first get past the gastric acids of the stomach and then are rapidly absorbed in the small intestine, whereas SCFAs are normally only produced in the large intestine by bacterial fermentation. The requirement for SCFAs to be at their natural site of production in the lumen of the large intestine, and at the correct concentrations, appears to be important for their effects on appetite regulation.[14]

However, if we cannot, for now, consume SCFAs as a supplement, the answer is then to keep our gut bacteria healthy with a wide variety of dietary fibre, and to also feed it with enough fermentable soluble fibre for it to produce just the right amount of SCFAs to keep us healthy. The easiest way to cultivate a happy and healthy (and wise?) microbiome is to eat a colourful selection of vegetables every day, for example, broccoli, carrots *and* tomatoes . . . and maybe throw in some aubergine (eggplant), which would give you four different colours!

FIBRE AND THE GLYCAEMIC INDEX OF FOOD

Another reason for the fabulousness of fibre is the fact that it reduces the caloric availability of foods. This is most clearly illustrated with the 'glycaemic index' of food. The glycaemic index or GI is a rating system used to show how quickly carbohydrate-containing foods affect blood glucose levels. It is, in effect, an indicator of the glucose availability of a given food. The original concept, although not by name, came from Dr George Campbell, one of Burkitt's influences in the development of the Fibre Hypothesis, who was interested in the role of dietary fibre in the development of type 2 diabetes. Stimulated by his interaction with Burkitt, Cleave and others, in 1969 Campbell embarked on a study of the blood-glucose response to carbohydrate digestion. Campbell recruited healthy volunteers and fed them 50 grams of carbohydrate from white or wholemeal bread, apples, corn starch, sucrose and glucose. He ranked the various carbohydrates according to the rise in blood glucose of the volunteers over time, and noted that the simple sugars were at the top of the list, while the starches and whole food were at the bottom. However, while Campbell did present this work at an international diabetes meeting in Amsterdam in 1971,[15] he never published it. So although these studies actually preceded, by a number of years, the better-known work of Phyllis Crapo in 1976 and David Jenkins in 1981, as with Burkitt and the fibre hypothesis above, most do not know of Campbell's role in the development of the glycaemic index. Crapo and her colleagues performed a series of studies comparing the effect of glucose, sucrose and starch, as well as potatoes and rice, on the blood-glucose levels of healthy adult subjects, and concluded that the more complex carbohydrates, such as starch, in food resulted in a lower blood-glucose and insulin response.[16] David Jenkins confirmed this phenomenon by performing similar studies on sixty-two commonly eaten foods and sugars, and was the one who actually coined the moniker 'glycaemic index'.[17]

More than forty years on, GI ratings have been compiled for many more than sixty-two different foods, and an entire 'GI Diet' has emerged. The highest GI food is, by definition, pure glucose. However, if any of you have ever tried it, glucose is actually oddly unpalatable, so while our body uses it as a primary fuel, we rarely ever consume it. The sugar we almost always use in food is sucrose, which is easily split into fructose and glucose, either by the acid in our stomach, or by the enzyme 'sucrase' that resides in the duodenum. Thus the glucose from sucrose is liberated with little effort and very quickly makes it into the bloodstream. The GI rating of sugar is therefore set at the maximum rating of 100, with all other foods indexed against that number. The principle of the GI Diet is to try and keep the rise in blood glucose after a meal as slow and steady as possible, by eating foods that take longer to digest and hence release their carbohydrates more slowly; so-called low-GI foods. The longer a particular food takes to digest . . . yup, you've got it, the further down the gut it will go before being absorbed, and the fuller you will feel. Low-GI foods are anything with a score of 55 or less, medium-GI foods 56 to 69, and high-GI foods will have a score above 70. Broadly speaking, the higher the GI of a food, the more rapidly it is digested, so you can't really discuss GI without considering caloric availability. As Campbell, Crapo and Jenkins all showed, the more complex the carbohydrate, the slower the rise in blood glucose. So starch does indeed have a lower GI than sucrose, but because it is made entirely from chains of glucose, not that much lower!

The key to keeping the GI rating of a particular food low? The all-important presence of fibre. For example, the GI rating for an orange is around 40, depending on its ripeness; it is considered 'low GI'. The GI rating for juice from that exact same orange, however, is more than 70! The fibre in an orange slows the release of the sugar from the orange juice. In the absence of fibre, however, the sugar, which incidentally is at the same concentration as that of a typical soda (and, yes, it is exactly the same sugar), is then absorbed with little digestion. Any foods that contain a lot of refined carbohydrates, either as free sugars or as refined white flour, or have very little fibre, are going to fall into the high-GI category. These are of course anything sugary, and also white bread, white rice and potatoes. Medium- and low-GI foods include some fruit and vegetables, pulses and whole grains, with the fibre and protein (in the pulses) slowing down their digestion.

So far so straightforward, until you take a closer peek at the many GI food lists and realise, perhaps unsurprisingly, that foods with a high GI are not necessarily unhealthy and not all foods with a low GI are healthy. The weakness of the GI rating system is that the GI is calculated based on a particular food being eaten in isolation. Case in point, cooking foods in fat or protein reduces the glucose availability, slowing down the absorption of carbohydrates and therefore lowering their GI. Potato crisps or chips or roast potatoes, for example, because they are cooked in fat, have a lower GI than boiled or baked potatoes. I adore all variations of potatoes that have been sympathetically introduced to hot fat . . . but, sadly, much as I wish it to be so, no one is going to say that a crisp or a roast potato is healthier than a boiled potato, thus they do have to be eaten in moderation.

The bottom line is, considering the GI of carbohydrate-containing foods is a great way to find healthier, higher-fibre and lower-sugar options. However, focusing only on the GI of foods, without taking into account other aspects, could result in an unbalanced diet, high in fat and calories, which could lead to weight gain, which was presumably not why you embarked upon this diet to begin with!

Aside from the GI diet, there are many other popular dietary approaches, some more rooted in science than others, that leverage the benefits of dietary fibre, particularly its influence on the caloric availability of food.

A PLANT-BASED APPROACH

Now returning to my newly minted role as the poster boy for the plant-based movement . . . Why did I lose weight after spending twenty-nine days on a plant-based diet? Plant-based foods (as opposed to crisps and faux bacon) are typically jam-packed full of fibre (plants being the primary source of dietary fibre) and so are bulkier and simply less calorically dense than meat, eggs or dairy. Simply put, because there are more calories per gram of animal-based food as compared to plant-based foods, you've gotta eat a lot of lentils and cabbage (other pulse–vegetable combinations are available) to match a plate of steak and eggs, and there is only so much time in the day for you to be chewing.

Additionally, the fibre in plant-based foods, as illustrated by the orange fruit versus orange juice example above, also reduces glucose availability and caloric availability more generally. Humans, as we have discussed, cannot digest most fibre and it just passes right through us. The calories present in most fibre are simply not 'available' for us to absorb. So even though I ate as much as I wanted during my meals, I was still absorbing fewer calories than if I had been eating animal-based food. On top of that, there would have been, presumably, raised levels of SCFAs produced by fermentation of the increased amounts of soluble fibre in my large intestine. To be clear, I didn't have my SCFA levels measured, but I can assure you I've never consumed that much fibre in all my life! The bottom line is this: the only way to lose weight is to eat less than you burn. The trick is to find an effective and sustainable way to do this that suits your own lifestyle and individual biology. For me, going vegan was clearly an effective way to absorb fewer calories, and hence I lost weight.

And how about my improved blood-cholesterol numbers? Part of the drop in my cholesterol levels could probably be explained by my weight loss, and part of it by the removal of saturated fat from my diet. Yes, I do realise that there are plant-based foods that are high in saturated fats – coconut milk is a case in point. However, for me, I know that the vast majority of the saturated fats that I was consuming would have come from meat or meat products.

Pork scratchings, you will recall from my visits to The Bell pub in the village I used to live in, are a particular weakness of mine, and of course so too are my favourite goose-fat roasted potatoes.

There are, however, two 'buts' (and they are very important buts) to consider. First, I would probably have seen the same effect had I switched to a low-dairy pescetarian diet. From the Italian word '*pesce*' for fish, this would mean that the bulk of animal-based protein in the diet would come from fish. While fish do contain fat, the vast proportion would be unsaturated fats. Eating unsaturated fats in place of saturated fats has been shown to reduce 'bad' LDL cholesterol, thus improving your cholesterol profile. Second, and most crucially, for many people, their cholesterol levels, because of their genetics, are not actually influenced by their diet at all. They can add or remove whatever they want from their diet and their cholesterol levels are not going to budge. So while a vegan diet had a positive effect on my cholesterol, this is not going to be true for everybody.

So with my poster-boy hat on, should you go plant-based? Well, it can be a healthy choice, as long as it is done with consideration and care. The most important thing to ensure when electing to shift to a vegan diet long-term is that it is nutritionally complete. This is generally not a problem if you are vegetarian, and are still eating dairy and eggs. If you are vegan, however, you have to ensure you are consuming enough protein, and make sure you get enough of certain micronutrients and fats.

Plant foods can definitely provide all of the protein we need, in particular the essential amino acids; these nutrients are protein building blocks that cannot be made by your body, and so have to be consumed. But it does depend on what you are eating. While skulking around supermarket aisles I found an item labelled 'vegan pulled pork'. Certain that it wasn't made using vegan pigs (it wasn't) and curious as to what was actually being 'pulled', I examined the package and read the small print. Aha, jackfruit, which is a tropical fruit from the fig family with a stringy consistency, was being used as a facsimile of pork. While ripe jackfruit has a sweet flavour profile somewhat akin to a cross between mango and pineapple, it has a neutral taste when it is unripe, making it ideal to absorb flavours, and it mimics meat surprisingly effectively. I have actually had jackfruit both as a fruit and in its guise as a 'meat', and it does taste great. The problem is, it contains a huge bolus of fibre, but next to no protein. So if you are having a 'vegan pulled pork' sandwich, and thinking you are having a complete meal, you are not! Good sources of plant-based protein are going to come from pulses – beans, lentils, chickpeas, tofu, soya alternatives to milk and yoghurt, or peanuts, for example – and from nuts (no, peanuts are not technically a 'nut').

In addition, there were also well-catalogued issues with micronutrient deficiencies in vegan diets to consider, in particular vitamin B12, which is found primarily in animal-based products. One of the notable exceptions is yeast extract, the source ingredient of Marmite (north of the equator) and Vegemite (south of the equator), which is vegan and does contain vitamin B12. However, the problem is that not everyone likes yeast extract; a 2011 YouGov poll put the UK 'I hate Marmite' camp at 33 per cent (with 33 per cent loving Marmite and 27 per cent not having an opinion either way).[18] What happens if you are a Marmite-hating vegan? Well, there is the option of 'nutritional yeast', which has a far more mellow taste than the concentrated extract, and is used almost as a seasoning. It's actually very tasty. Regardless, because vitamin B12 is essential for health, including maintaining a properly functioning brain and sufficient red blood cells, those on a long-term vegan diet, whatever their views on Marmite, are recommended to take a B12 supplement.

Iodine is something else that vegans need to be careful they get enough of. It is essential for the production of thyroid hormone, which plays an important role in growth and metabolism in humans. While seafood is a famously rich source of iodine, most people in the UK and in the US actually get much of their iodine from dairy products. It's not that cows are intrinsically high in iodine, per se; rather, their feed is, and this iodine makes it into the milk. So where should vegans be getting their iodine from? Seaweed is a very useful source, but aside for vegan sushi and sometimes in (non-instant) ramen, it is not a major food source in this country. While there are other plant-based sources of iodine, such as potatoes or corn or strawberries, for instance, the levels contained are really quite low. Thus, like with B12, vegans are advised to include an iodine supplement in their diet.

Finally, there are a couple of fats classed as essential because our bodies cannot make them. The essential omega-3 and omega-6 fats are crucial for the healthy functioning of our immune system, brain, nerves and eyes. Omega 3 and 6 famously come from fish, but you can also get them from various seeds, walnuts, soy and avocados.

FLEXITARIAN

Thus it was that on a cold afternoon in April a lighter and lower-cholesterol me left the University of Coventry with a spring in my step. At the train station, I celebrated with a bag of non-vegan 'cheese and onion' crisps. Although on closer examination of the ingredient list, the amount of actual 'cheese' that was present in the bag was vanishingly small . . . almost homeopathic in its dose. But it didn't matter! Psychologically, to me it felt like I was consuming a whole chunk of mature Cheddar cheese or blue Stilton.

That evening, because it just happened to be a Friday, I went to my local curry house, and for the first time in four weeks I could order my favourite king prawn curry with egg pilau rice and naan bread. The first bite into a mouthful of prawn jalfrezi lit up every reward circuit in my brain like a Christmas tree ... or that was certainly what it felt like! And then I had dairy ice-cream after, just because I could. On Saturday I had a steak, on Sunday I had sausages and eggs for breakfast and for dinner, roast pork, served with crackling and goose fat-roasted potatoes.

Then very rapidly, two things happened. First, after a weekend of post-vegan hedonistic animal-based feasting, there were complaints from my guts and their bacterial denizens, and I can tell you that it wasn't pleasant. They had clearly got used to being bathed in lovely fibre-rich plant-based food, even after only four weeks. Second, I gained 2 kilograms, or 5 pounds, in weight within five days of coming off the vegan diet. That is half the weight that it took me four weeks to lose, back in five days, and I'm almost certain it was ALL fat. Diets only work if you are actually on the diet. When I stopped being vegan, the caloric density of the food I was eating had changed so drastically that the weight was simply flooding back. It was then I made the decision. I knew that I had to fundamentally change something in my life, as I was determined not to waste all of the hard work and all of the health gains.

So I changed my eating behaviour as a result of this experiment. While I missed meat too much to give it up entirely, I took the route of compromise and moderation (rare these days) and became a 'flexitarian', whereby I am vegan during weekday lunches and at least twice a week in the evenings. That might seem like a cop-out to some, but I have probably cut my meat intake by 40 to 50 per cent, and that can only be a good thing. To me, cooking vegan food was no longer this scary thing, and I no longer considered it an inferior-quality product. Crucially, this dietary change was, for me, sustainable. Coupled with the addition of some resistance training to my daily cycling regime, I have managed to get back down to my vegan fighting weight, and have maintained the lighter me for the past three years and counting. I can't overstate to you that given my love of meat, how unlikely an outcome this would have seemed before I started this whole adventure. If you don't believe me, ask my wife! She was, and is still, stunned by my change in behaviour. What is it they say about an old dog and spots, and leopards and tricks?

MEDITERRANEAN LIVING

In most Chinese households, mine included, you will find the statues of three old men placed in some prominent position. In our house (my wife finds them a bit kitsch – frankly, they are – and is not a fan, but she allows me this cultural luxury) they have pride of place in the living room, next to our TV. These are the Sanxing 三星 or 'Three Stars' Chinese deities that date from the Ming dynasty, Fu 福, Lu 禄, and Shou 寿. Fu for good fortune, Lu representing prosperity, and Shou meaning longevity, the three attributes that Chinese culture (and many others too, I'm sure) considers to be central to a good life. Longevity, in particular, is universally aspired to, and there are certain regions in the world where the local populations famously have a greater longevity than others. The Japanese on the island of Okinawa and Costa Ricans living on the Nicoya Peninsula are classic examples, and there is great interest in understanding why this might be the case. Genetics will undoubtedly have a large say, but the diets of these people are also the subject of scrutiny. One other important group notable for their health and longer lifespans is those living along the shores of the Mediterranean, and in recent years, considerable efforts have been put into studying the benefits of their diet.

The traditional Mediterranean diet is characterized by a high intake of olive oil, nuts, fruit, vegetables, grains and cereals. It encourages a moderate intake of fish and poultry and a low intake of dairy products, red meat, processed meats, and sweets. Finally (and most importantly?), wine can be consumed in moderation, but with meals. Many observational studies have shown that risk of cardiovascular disease goes down with adherence to a Mediterranean diet. Crucially, there was a large randomised trial performed by Spanish scientists to test the effectiveness of two variations of the Mediterranean diets, one supplemented with extra-virgin olive oil and another with nuts, as compared with a low-fat control diet combined with dietary advice.[19] What they found was that folks on either the extra-virgin olive oil or nut versions of the Mediterranean diet had a 30 per cent reduction in major cardiovascular events compared to those on the regular 'low-fat' diet! Thirty per cent! Keep in mind that cardiovascular disease remains the most common cause of death in the world, accounting for 31 per cent of ALL deaths in 2017.[20] These numbers are also likely to be an underestimate of the effectiveness of the diet, because it was compared against people on a low-fat diet and provided with support, as opposed to being fed an unhealthy diet. Why? Because ethically you cannot recruit people at high risk of heart and metabolic disease for a trial and proceed to feed them doughnuts! Last time I checked, that would be frowned upon. The really interesting thing in this case was that the key driver in protecting against heart disease did not appear to be weight loss (although weight loss would have independent protective effects), because there were no significant weight differences between the groups. Rather, it did appear to be the Mediterranean diet per se.

So what exactly is it about the Mediterranean diet that is beneficial? People being people, they want to know, presumably so they can put it into a pill and sell it as a supplement. Is it the flavonoids in the olive oil? The reduction in red and processed meats? The reduction in saturated fats and the increase in unsaturated fats? Or the increased dietary fibre as a result of copious consumption of fruit, vegetables and whole grains? Surely the answer is most likely to be 'all of the above'!

RAW

Then we get to the diets on the other end of the scientific (or lack thereof) spectrum. Take the 'raw' movement, for example. Raw foodies define 'raw food' as anything that has not been refined, canned or chemically processed, and has not been heated above 48°C. The claim is that by heating food the natural enzymes are destroyed, so the body has to work harder in order to produce more of its own enzymes, exhausting its energy. Wow . . . can I use emojis in response here? A picture and a thousand words and all that. First, cooking will not only destroy some of the natural enzymes in food (as opposed to, I guess, unnatural enzymes in your food?), it will destroy pretty much all of the enzymes in the food. Even if you did eat a raw apple or a carrot, the acid in your stomach would do a pretty number on destroying those natural enzymes anyway. Whatever hardy enzymes do survive that acidic cauldron of the stomach will then be fully digested in the small intestines before being absorbed into our system. When we eat another plant or animal, everything is broken down into its constituent parts and reassembled in each cell into human proteins and enzymes and everything else, according to the instructions written in our genes. I can't believe it needs to be said, but eating an antelope won't make us run any faster, neither will eating a duck or any other bird make you able to fly. We just can't co-opt the enzymes from a cow, or salmon, or for that matter broccoli, to use in our own bodies. That is simply not how biology works. Cooking does indeed destroy some heat-sensitive micronutrients such as vitamin C, for example. We get around that by eating much of our fruit, and some of our vegetables, which are of course rich in vitamin C, raw. This is undoubtedly something we don't do enough of and is to be encouraged.

Raw food, which, aside from sushi and beef tartare is going to be plant-based, is of course packed full of fibre. Eating raw food – a salad, basically – means you will be absorbing far fewer calories, which is why a raw-food diet is so effective for weight loss. Cooking, after all, increases the caloric availability of food. It of course also kills most parasites that might be present in the food, which surely is a good thing . . . otherwise you might end up losing weight for entirely the wrong reason!

SIRTFOOD DIET

Early in 2020, the singer Adele reappeared in public after months of radio silence, on the occasion of her thirty-second birthday, and shocked everyone by having dropped 100 pounds in weight.[21] I am a fan, and she was, indeed, almost unrecognisable. All of the newspapers, celebrity magazines and online tabloids breathlessly reported on her 'miraculous' weight loss; people, from A-listers to regular Joes and Janets, all gushed about how amazing she now looked. I found the response fascinating. Did she not look amazing before? Is she now more of a woman because there is less of her? Also, as a scientist who is government funded to tackle the crisis of obesity, and I don't think using the word crisis is hyperbole, should I not also be celebrating Adele's reduction in body size? If Adele, or anyone else for that matter, chooses to and successfully loses weight, whatever the reasons, all power to her or them. There will be undoubted health benefits in doing so. The problem I have with this whole scenario is that by fetishising someone else's weight loss, by framing its success as a triumph over previously bad choices, then, by default, those that fail to lose the weight are deemed to be continuing to make bad choices. But many many people, for a myriad of different reasons, will always find weight loss like this close to impossible. They are not bad people, they are, instead fighting both their biology and their personal circumstance. Anyway, end of editorial interlude, and we now return to your regularly scheduled programming.

Adele's weight loss, as reported by everyone, was all thanks to the newest of new fads, the Sirtfood Diet[22]. Developed by two British nutritionists, Aidan Goggins and Glen Matten, the diet is called Sirt because it is based on eating foods that, apparently, activate the sirtuin proteins in the body. There are seven members to the sirtuin family, and it is true that each play various roles in regulating metabolism, inflammation and the longevity of cells. Activating these proteins then leads, according to Goggins and Matten, to the turning on of your 'skinny gene'. They, of course, have written a book that is the 'official' guide, *The Official Sirtfood Diet*.[23] One of the selling points to the diet is that it allows red wine and chocolate which, I must admit, is undoubtedly appealing.

The diet combines sirtfoods and calorie restriction, which is what activates the sirtuins. Right, I'm now going to stop trying to explain any more of the 'science' behind the diet, because it is killing trees and not explaining how the diet actually works . . . and it undoubtedly worked for Adele! First, the Sirtfood Diet includes an explicit reference to calorie restriction, which is hardly a unique dietary strategy. Then, if we have a look at the top twenty sirtfoods they include kale, red wine, strawberries, onions, soy, parsley, extra-virgin olive oil, dark chocolate (85 per cent cocoa), matcha green tea, buckwheat, turmeric, walnuts, rocket, bird's eye chilli, lovage, medjool dates, red chicory, blueberries, capers and coffee. What leaps out immediately? Well, for one thing, it appears oddly specific. Bird's eye chillis? How about habanero or jalapeños or scotch bonnets? Medjool dates? How about barhee or halawi or safawi dates? I am always deeply suspicious of diets (as opposed to recipes) that list very specific types of food – the more to restrict you with, my dear. More importantly, it is clear that sirtfoods are largely, if not entirely (although I have not done an extensive survey) plant-based.

Need I say more? The sirtfood diet is nothing more than a plant-based diet (which we now know works as a weight-loss strategy for some), coupled with calorie restriction, wrapped up in some 'sciency' explanation to make it more compelling.

ALKALINE LIVING

While the Sirtfood Diet is one of the new kids on the block, the playbook that it uses, of producing a list of foods that you should or should not eat, and packaging it with a convoluted explanation, is as old as time. Just look at the wide variety of food restrictions that are linked with different religions, including the major monotheistic faiths. In many ways, given the evangelical fervour with which many follow, promote and/or defend different dietary approaches, the way we eat appears to have been transformed in the twenty-first century into yet another form of religion. Some of these new religions, these new diets, have more complicated and convoluted playbooks than others, none more so than the Alkaline Diet.

In 2002, Robert Young published the book *The pH Miracle* that touched on the alkaline movement.[24] The basis for the Alkaline Diet is this: because our blood is pH 7.4, which is slightly alkali (pH 7.0 is neutral, with anything below 7 being acidic and anything above 7 being alkali), we therefore need to eat alkalising foods, as opposed to acidic foods, in order to maintain our blood pH and our health. Nothing could be simpler, right? The trick, of course, is to know what foods are alkalising and what foods are acidic. Of course, *The pH Miracle* helpfully provides colourful and detailed charts of appropriately alkali foods in which you are encouraged to indulge, and terrible acidic foods you should avoid like the plague.

Now, whatever you might think about gluten-free or plant-based, at the very least the names actually describe the diet. Anyone who chooses to follow the diet can do so easily; they may be restrictive, but the rules are simple. The problem with the Alkali Diet is that whether a food has been designated as acid or alkalising has little to do with the actual pH of those foods. The most egregious example is that lemons and limes are listed as alkalising, and thus are good for you. There is little doubt that lemons and limes, packed as they are with vitamin C and other nutritional goodies, are fabulous for one's diet. The problem is that vitamin C is known as ascorbic *acid*, and lemons and limes, which are citrus fruits after all, contain citric *acid*. In fact, lemon juice actually has a very acidic pH of 2. Another example is that, according to *The pH Miracle*, most foods get more acidic when cooked, so it is better to eat food raw, or minimally cooked and in their 'natural' state. Raw unpasteurised milk, for instance, is supposed to be neutral in pH, but becomes acidic when pasteurised. So drink raw! Milk is indeed slightly acidic with a pH of 6.5, because of lactose being converted to lactic acid. But it is pH 6.5 whether or not it has been heated as part of the pasteurisation process; it doesn't change. Incidentally, the US Centre for Disease Control (CDC) says that improperly handled raw milk is responsible for nearly three times more hospitalisations than any other food-borne disease source, making it one of the world's most dangerous food products. Hurrah for pasteurisation! Bottom line, there is no rationale, certainly based on any science that I know of, for why *The pH Miracle* categorises foods as acid or alkali, even if by chance they sometimes get it right; it is almost entirely made up.

Let's just say that you could somehow bring yourself to accept Robert Young's alkali and acidic food taxonomy, the whole concept of the Alkali Diet still tumbles down because it ignores the presence of the stomach, which at pH 1.5 is by some distance the most acidic compartment in our body. As we discuss in Chapter 3, anything you eat, whatever its actual (or even fantastical) starting pH, will be thoroughly acidified by the gastric juices in the stomach before moving into the duodenum of the small intestine, where it is neutralised. Nothing we eat can change the pH of our blood.

In spite of its nonsensical nature, barely able to stand up to casual scrutiny, the Alkali Diet remains as popular as ever, with many celebrities embracing the alkali way, including seven-time Superbowl-winning quarterback Tom Brady.[25] The only reason it continues to attract so many followers is probably because it works for weight loss. Why? As it turns out, because meat and most other animal-based products are labelled as 'acidic', an alkali diet is pretty much a plant-based diet by another name. So at the risk of sounding like a broken record, plant-based, fibre, caloric availability, blah blah blah.

FABULOUS FIBRE

So all of these dietary approaches that we have discussed, and many more that we haven't, are in fact largely vegetarian or plant-based diets by another name, which leverage the health benefits of fabulous fibre but with far more complicated rules. Why not just sell a vegetarian or plant-based cookbook or website or television programme? Perhaps I'm being cynical here, but in a very crowded space, I can't help but think that these are just marketing ploys. Also, to be honest, openly declaring a book to be vegetarian or vegan or plant-based would probably put off a significant proportion of the population, and that is a legitimate issue to address and discuss. In the meantime, whatever motivates you and works for you, be it Raw, or Sirt or Alkali or anything else that isn't dangerous, then you do you. But please don't foist your choices that you are privileged enough to make on others, and spare me the pseudo-scientific mumbo jumbo about activating sirtuins and skinny genes, or alkalising your blood with lemon juice.

CHAPTER 7

The 'ultra' in processed

It was early morning in January, just gone 6 a.m., when we arrived at a dairy farm in Reading, England. As I opened the car door, the cold air hit me, pungent with the aroma of cattle, making me catch my breath. It was still dark, but the lights from within the large building in front of us dimly illuminated the yard, just enough for me to see light snow falling. The ground was a sloppy and muddy mess. Katie, one of the producers who had driven us there, handed me a pair of Wellington boots.

'I got these from the props department, so they may not be the right size, but at least you won't smell like cows for the rest of the day.'

I put them on and they were too big. It made me feel like I had clown's feet, but at least I wouldn't smell like cows for the rest of the day! I pulled on a beanie and a pair of gloves, hopped out of the car and squelched across the yard to where we were greeted by the farmer, Andy, who was wearing some professional-looking and well-worn wellies that actually fitted. He took us into the large facility. To the right we could see, smell and hear more than a hundred cows, munching on hay (but of course they chew, swallow, unswallow and rechew ... so they are probably constantly chewing) and mooing in a bovine fashion.

'They're already done for the morning. We've left a few cows unmilked so that you could film the process.'

The clear unspoken implication was that we were late. It wasn't even 6.30 a.m. and most of the milking had already been done? Gosh, these farmers don't mess about.

The automated milking facility could accommodate up to twenty cows at once, in two rows of ten, on a slightly raised grated stainless-steel platform, with a lowered pit area in between. We heard a voice yelling:

'Go on, girls, move on in! Come on, move on in!'

Then ten surprisingly (to me at any rate) large beasts entered the right-hand side platform in a row, placidly walking up to the milking stations, and then each reversing slightly until their backsides were pressed up against the metal cages. It was all performed with impressive synchronisation and precision. They had clearly done this before. I was invited by one of the workers (would he have been a cowboy?) down into the pit. He began to clean the udders and teats of the cows, which, once you were down there, were at eye level. I had certainly never been quite this close to a cow before, let alone from this particular vantage point. We seemed perilously close to the, shall we say, 'business end'. Andy caught me looking up in some trepidation and yelled above the mooing:

'Yes, do watch out, the ladies sometimes get a bit excited when they are being milked!'

Oh fabulous, I thought to myself. How exactly were my poorly fitting wellies going to help if that happened?

At this point, the automated milking devices at the respective stations whirred into action. Each had four tubes topped with suction cups and was controlled remotely by the farmer. First some green disinfectant came bubbling out of each of the tubes and was then quickly washed away. Once all traces of green were gone, the cowboy who was down with me in the pit began to attach the milking tubes to each cow. The pumps then whirred into action, and milk began to travel from the tubes up into stainless steel pipes above the platform, which led away from the building into some unseen giant receptacle. Each Holstein Friesian produces around ten thousand litres of milk a year. They are milked twice a day, every day, so 13 to 14 litres of milk emerges from each cow during each milking session. This particular farm had 200 head of cattle, which meant more than 5,000 litres of raw milk was produced a day.

I was at the farm that morning for the BBC's *Trust Me, I'm a Doctor* series to film a piece about the nutritional benefits of cow's milk versus the ever-increasing proliferation of various non-dairy milk substitutes. All of the milk we get from the supermarket and shops today is pasteurised, so milk is actually a 'processed food'. Most of the plant-based milk options, with the exception of co-conut milk, because of all the machinations that are required to convert quinoa or oat extract into a facsimile of milk (how exactly do you milk a quinoa?), are actually classed as 'ultra-processed'. While these milk replacements are ideal for those on a vegan or plant-based diet, as well as lactose-intolerant folks such as myself, they are, in most high-income countries, targeted primarily at the rapidly growing health and wellness market.

Here's the interesting thing, though, the term 'ultra-processed' has, in recent years, been synonymous with unhealthy fast-food options, high in sugar, fat and salt, that are blamed for the obeso-genic environment we find ourselves in today. Ultra-processed food is the opposite of 'clean', the antithesis of 'real'. Yet ultra-processed plant-based milks are unashamedly marketed as healthy. What makes one ultra-processed food item different from another? What makes some suited to be condemned and legislat-ed against, while others remain respectable, eminently Instagram-mable, even?

WHAT MAKES A FOOD PROCESSED?

Heat

The term 'processed' is a broad church. Cooking, for example, the primal act of applying heat to food, is by definition a 'process'. The pioneering humans who first stuck a piece of antelope or a proto-potato onto a stick and waved it over a flame must have thought, *gosh, this smells a lot better after its been heated through . . . who knew BBQ'd venison and a baked potato could taste so good?* Aroma and taste aside, cooking crucially sterilised food of pesky parasites and increased its caloric availability, providing an increased number of calories for the same amount of work. Today, there are a gazillion fancy-shmancy ways to cook our food of course, *sous vide* (sealed and in a water bath), *en papillote* (wrapped in paper in the oven), blow-torched (an unnecessarily dangerous cooking implement) . . . but at its essence, cooking is still simply applying heat to food.

Heat can also be used as part of the process of preservation. Pasteurisation, for instance, heats milk (and other types of liquid) up to 60°C to 72°C for a few seconds, killing off the majority of microbes without impairing flavour, and extending the shelf life of milk from a couple of days to two weeks or more in the fridge. Improperly handled raw milk is actually one of the world's most dangerous causes of food poisoning. In contrast, the far less nuanced approach of blasting milk with 135°C heat for a few seconds – sterilising it, essentially – produces ultra-high-temperature treated (UHT) milk, which extends the life of milk, if correctly sealed, to months at room temperature. However, the high heat denatures some of the protein in the milk and ends up impairing its flavour. My wife, Jane, who you will recall is a 'cuppa tea' aficionado, cannot abide UHT milk in tea as it ruins the flavour, or so she (and many other English folk) says. Fresh (meaning pasteurised) milk only, she says! I wouldn't know as I'm lactose in-tolerant! Finally, putting food, just cooked and still piping hot, into a heat-sterilised container and then sealing it, as happens during the canning process or when one is making jam, extends its shelf life indefinitely, often without the use of any preservatives.

Salt, sugar and smoke

In fact, prior to the advent of refrigeration, the primary reason for most food processing was for the purpose of preservation. The curing of meat and fish is probably the oldest such example, and has been a dominant method of food preservation for thousands of years. Meat or fish were most commonly cured by the addition of salt or, when it became available, sugar, with the aim of drawing moisture out of the food by the process of osmosis. The result-ing decrease in moisture content and increase of salt and/or sugar concentration within the meat or fish discouraged the growth of bacteria and other microorganisms that cause food to spoil. Often, smoking is also performed together with salt curing, which seals the outer layer of the food being cured, making it more dif-ficult for bacteria to enter. Thus emerged bacon and ham (both smoked and unsmoked), beef jerky and smoked fish, including salmon, haddock and mackerel. Dehydration, by simply drying food out in the sun, is another of the earliest forms of food preser-vation and works because bacterial growth requires water. Fruit is often preserved in this way, such as sun-dried tomatoes, prunes, raisins, dried apricots and dried dates, as are mushrooms, includ-ing dried porcini and shitakes.

Fermentation

Then there is harnessing the process of fermentation by micro-organisms as a method of food preservation. The earliest docu-mented use of fermentation dates back to nearly 7000BC in Jiahu, China, where the first evidence of an alcoholic drink made from the fermentation of fruit was discovered. Yogurt, which is produced by the bacterial fermentation of milk, converting lactose to lactic acid, was thought to have been invented in Mesopotamia around 5000BC. Fermentation has also been used as a method of preserving vegetables in many cultures, with examples of fermented cabbage that include sauerkraut in Europe and kimchi in Korea, and also used to create condiments including soy sauce, and fermented yellow and black soy beans.

Treatment of grains

What will surprise many is that the grains that we eat every day, from which humans get the majority of their calories, are also processed. Rice and wheat, for example, have been milled, which is where the husk, bran and germ are removed. The act of polishing after milling is what gives rice its characteristic white colour, and its taste and texture. Crucially this refining of rice extended the storage life of the dried grain, which would presumably have been the primary reason why it was developed. There is also another process, developed and practised by indigenous peoples in the Americas, of soaking corn in an alkaline solution, typically lime (not the fruit but the mineral), prior to cooking. The problem with corn is that while it is particularly rich in the micronutrient niacin, otherwise known as vitamin B_3, the niacin is chemically unavailable to the human digestive system, and so would pass right through us. Soaking the corn in an alkaline solution liberated the niacin, making it available to us during digestion. How the indigenous Americans worked this out is a mystery but seeing as corn was domesticated some 10,000 years ago, work it out through trial and error they did.

So while the term 'processed food', as used today, is associated with a whole host of negative connotations, the processes of cooking, food preservation and separation were critical to our ability as a species to survive and to thrive; they reduced the chances of food poisoning, increased caloric availability, ensured that we had a predictable source of calories through seasonal changes in the availability of fresh food, and buffered against environmental crises such as drought.

WHAT MAKES PROCESSED FOODS 'ULTRA'?

However, while the processing of food is as ancient as human-kind, contemporary methods of industrial processing have led to so-called 'ultra-processed' foods. According to the Merriam-Webster dictionary, the prefix 'ultra' can mean 'beyond in space' or 'on the other side', such as in ultraviolet; it can mean 'beyond the limits of' or 'transcending'; or it can mean 'beyond what is or-dinary, proper, or moderate'. It is this last usage that reflects what many today think about this most modern of phenomena, foods that have been processed beyond what is ordinary or proper.

The concept of ultra-processed foods was first mooted by Pro-fessor Carlos Monteiro, director of the Centre for Epidemiologic-al Studies in Health and Nutrition at the University of Sao Paulo in Brazil, in a commentary written in 2009. In it, Monteiro argues that:

'The issue is not food, nor nutrients, so much as processing,' and that '[f]rom the point of view of human health, at present, the most salient division of foods and drinks is in terms of their type, degree and purpose of processing.'[1]

The idea was developed and discussed over the next few years, and then in early 2016, Monteiro and his colleagues proposed a new system to classify foods and food products based on the extent and purpose of the industrial processes applied to preserve, extract, modify or create them. They called this the NOVA (a name and not an acronym) system of food classification.[2]

NOVA divides foods into four different groups:

Group 1 – Unprocessed or minimally processed foods

This first group includes obviously unprocessed foods such as fresh fruits and vegetables, fresh or frozen meat and fish, and eggs. It also includes foods that have been minimally processed, which include the removal of inedible or unwanted parts, drying, crushing, grinding, fractioning, filtering, roasting, boiling, pasteurisation, refrigeration, freezing, placing in containers, vacuum packaging or non-alcoholic fermentation. None of these processes adds salt, sugar, oils, fats or other substances to the original food. The purposes of these processes are to extend the life of unprocessed foods, allowing their storage for longer use, as well as to facilitate food preparation, such as in the crushing or grinding of seeds and the roasting of coffee beans or drying of tea leaves.

Group 2 – Processed culinary ingredients

This second group encompasses processed ingredients extracted either directly from Group 1 foods, or from nature, by processes such as pressing, refining, grinding, milling and drying. It includes, for example, purifying salt from seawater; extracting sugar from cane or beet; removing honey from combs and syrup from maple trees; extracting vegetable oils by crushing olives or seeds; producing butter from milk; and extracting starches from corn and other plants. These Group 2 ingredients tend to be used to prepare, season and cook Group 1 foods and to make them more varied and enjoyable. They also include products such as salted butter, iodised salt, and vinegar made by acetic fermentation of wine or other alcoholic drinks. Group 2 items are rarely consumed in the absence of Group 1 foods.

Group 3 – Processed foods

The third NOVA group comprises processed foods. These products could be made by adding sugar, oil, salt or other Group 2 substances to Group 1 foods, for instance. Processes include various preservation or cooking methods, and, in the case of breads and cheeses, non-alcoholic fermentation. The main purpose of the manufacture of processed foods is to increase the shelf-life of Group 1 foods; very often these processes end up modifying or enhancing the taste, texture and smell of the foods. Typical processed foods include canned or bottled vegetables, fruits and legumes; salted or sugared nuts and seeds; salted, cured, or smoked meats; canned fish; fruits in syrup; cheeses and unpackaged freshly made breads. These foods may contain additives used for preservation and to resist microbial contamination, and include fruits in syrup with added antioxidants, and cured meats with added preservatives. Alcoholic drinks that are produced by fermentation of Group 1 foods, such as beer, cider and wine, are included here in Group 3.

Group 4 – Ultra-processed food and drink products
And then we have the all-important Group 4; it is here that all of the ultra-processed food and drink products reside. As defined by Monteiro, ultra-processed foods are, in effect, industrial formulations, typically with five or usually many more ingredients that most would find difficult, if not impossible, to replicate in a domestic situation. These foods contain substances not commonly used, if at all, in normal restaurant or home cooking. Ingredients only found in ultra-processed products include some that are directly extracted from foods, such as gluten and the milk derivatives of casein, lactose and whey, while others result from further processing of food constituents, and include products such as hydrogenated or interesterified oils, hydrolysed proteins, maltodextrin and high-fructose corn syrup. They can also contain additives – such as dyes, colour stabilisers, flavourings and other flavour enhancers and artificial sweeteners – and processing aids such as emulsifiers, and carbonating, bulking and anti-caking agents. Other methods used in the manufacture of ultra-processed

foods include industrial-scale extrusion and moulding, which is a long way from using a jelly mould or a domestic pasta-making machine.

Just to list a few examples, ultra-processed products are pretty much all carbonated drinks; any sweet or savoury packaged snacks and confectionery; ice-cream (right, I quit now); mass-produced packaged breads and buns; cookies or biscuits (depending where in the world you are from); margarines and spreads; pastries, cakes and cake mixes; breakfast 'cereals'; meat extracts and bouillon cubes; infant formulas, follow-on milks and other baby products; many ready-to-heat meals including pre-prepared pies and pasta and pizzas; chicken nuggets, fish fingers, sausages, burgers and hot dogs made from reconstituted meat products; and 'instant' noodles (right, I quit for a second time in a paragraph) and desserts. And many many other items.

Then here is the tricky thing. There are foods that appear to be from either Groups 1 or 3, but because they contain additives become classed as Group 4. So plain yoghurt is a Group 1 food, however, if flavourings, or sugar, or artificial sweeteners, or sweetened granola are added, it becomes Group 4; it becomes ultra-processed. Bread is a processed food, but if made with added emulsifiers and gluten, it becomes ultra-processed. Also, while alcoholic drinks made by fermentation are processed, their further distillation into whisky, gin, rum or vodka transforms them into an ultra-processed product.

Of these, Monteiro had this to say:

'Diets that include a lot of ultra-processed foods are intrinsically nutritionally unbalanced and intrinsically harmful to health.'[3]

Sounds deeply depressing, I know.

THE MORE ULTRA-PROCESSED FOOD WE
EAT, THE HEAVIER WE GET

The problem is, we LOVE our ultra-processed goodies! God help the person that comes between me and a pre-packaged loaf of brioche bread, or ice-cream, or sometimes both together (try it: a scoop of double chocolate fudge ice-cream on a slice of just toasted and still warm brioche – you'll thank me later).

How much do we love these foods? Well, in 2016, the top three countries in the world for the consumption of ultra-processed foods were all in Europe.[4] Top of the pile is the Netherlands, who consumed 143.8 kilograms per person per year; then we have Germany at 141.8 kilograms per person per year; and then the UK at 140.7 kilograms per person per year; fourth is Norway (128.8): fifth Finland (124.6); sixth Ireland (124.2); seventh New Zealand (115.9); and a surprising eighth, the USA (115.8). The USA do lead the world in ultra-processed drinks, though, at 238.8 kilograms per person per year (because 1 kilogram of water = 1 litre of water, that is near enough 238.8 litres per person per year), swiftly followed by Mexico in second at 188.5 litres per person per year, and then Argentina in third at 184.5 litres per person per year. The UK is all the way down at sixteenth with 124.4 litres per person per year; it must be all the hot tea (unprocessed) that is drunk instead.

Let's just reflect for a minute on what these numbers actually entail. In the UK, where I live, we consume 140 kilograms of ultra-processed food and 124.4 litres of ultra-processed drink per person per year, or 0.39 kilograms of food and 0.34 litres of drink every single day, on average. That is, to put it into a more familiar context, equivalent to 7.7 Mars bars (other ultra-processed bar-shaped cocoa-based confectioneries are available) and a can of soda every day. If we look at the USA, they consume 115.8 kilograms of ultra-processed food and a whopping 238.8 litres of ultra-processed drink per person per year. That is 0.32 kilograms of food and 0.65 litres of drink every single day, on average. So while consuming a little less ultra-processed food, Americans drink nearly twice the amount of ultra-processed drink. Anyone who has had the fortune to visit the 7-Eleven chain of US corner shops for one of their 'big-gulp'-sized drinks, which come with up to 50 fluid ounces or 1.48 litres of your favourite carbonated beverage, can see how one can easily consume 0.65 litres of ultra-processed drink a day. In fact, more than 50 per cent of our calories, at least in Europe, Australia, New Zealand and North America, come from ultra-processed foods. The numbers are even more scary for kids, with 65 per cent of calories eaten by primary and secondary-school children in the UK, for example, coming from ultra-processed food or drinks.[5] Yup, you heard that right . . . 65 per cent!

At the other end of the spectrum, in 2016 we have Cameroon consuming 1.9 kilograms per person per year of ultra-processed food, Pakistan on 3.6 kilograms per person per year and India on 3.8 kilograms per person per year. As for drinks, India consumes 5.7 litres per person per year, Kenya 9.9 litres per person per year and Pakistan 10 litres per person per year. The difference between the top and bottom of the scale is stark. However, ultra-processed food and drink sales per capita increased everywhere from 2002 to 2016, except in Western Europe, North America, and Australasia, which have demonstrated slight decreases, but from astronomically high starting points. Pakistan and India, for instance, have more than doubled their consumption, per person, of ultra-processed foods between 2002 and 2016, going from a low baseline of 1.5 kilograms per person per year to 3.6 kilograms and 3.8 kilograms per person per year respectively.[6]

Studies conducted in Europe between 1991 and 2008 showed that the average household availability of ultra-processed food and drink ranged from around 10 per cent of total purchased calories in Portugal to just over 50 per cent in the UK.[7] While accepting that comparing food consumption practices between different countries is fraught with confounding factors, even after taking these into account, each per-cent increase in the availability of ultra-processed calories in an average household was associated with an increase of 0.25 per cent in obesity prevalence within that country. This association is not confined to Europe, of course. In Latin America, sales of ultra-processed food and drink have also been linked with weight gain, with each 20 kilogram per person per year increase associated with an increase of 0.28 on average BMI (weight in kilograms divided by height in metres squared).[8] In fact, taking into account all the regions of the world, for every 51 litres per person per year in ultra-processed drink volume sales, average BMI increased by 0.195 kilograms per metre squared in men and 0.072 kilograms per metre squared for women. And for every 40 kilogram per person per year in ultra-processed food sales, average BMI increased by 0.316 kilograms per metre squared for men, whereas the association was not significant for women.[9] Women, once again proving to be the superior half of humanity, clearly drink less soda and eat less junk! These numbers might seem small, but remember that these are population-level averages, and these small increases translate to a lot of people getting much larger.

'RECONSTITUTED PROTEIN OF ANIMAL ORIGIN'

However, keep in mind that there is a broad spectrum of just how processed an ultra-processed product is; ranging from adding a sweetener to a yoghurt or emulsifier and gluten to bread, to the use of centrifuged or mechanically reconstituted protein of animal origin.

You say what now?

(Warning: vegetarians and vegans look away now.)

There are a number of industrial processes that are used to extract every iota of meat from the bones, once the prime cuts have been removed. Take, for example, a highly processed and widely used beef product, which has been pejoratively referred to as 'pink slime' (I'm no PR guru, but it is something I would not recommend including in the marketing material), euphemistically labelled as 'lean finely textured beef'. This is produced by heating the last traces of meat and other bits that have been scraped off the carcass in order to melt the fat, which is then removed by centrifugation or spinning at high-speed; the pink-coloured fat-depleted 'meat' (hence the moniker 'pink slime') is then either treated with ammonium hydroxide gas or citric acid to kill any bacteria, and the resulting product is pressed and frozen. This product is currently not allowed for human consumption in Canada or the EU. In the US, 'lean finely textured beef' is not sold directly to the consumer; it looks like pink soft-serve ice-cream but is actually beef paste (yum!) . . . trust me, even if it were available for purchase, no one would buy it. Rather, it can constitute up to 15 per cent of some mince-beef items without additional labelling. So the fancy steak mince that you or I might buy for homemade burgers, meatballs or pasta sauce, is just that; a piece of meat that has been ground up, and typically ranges in fat content from 5 to 15 per cent. However, manufacturers sometimes use cheaper, and hence fattier, cuts to make minced beef, which pushes the fat content up to 30 to 35 per cent, and that doesn't look so good on the front-of-pack labelling. So by adding in lean finely textured beef they can reduce the total fat content of the product. This tactic is used in items such as certain varieties of frozen burger patties and other processed beef products.

Then there is 'mechanically separated poultry', where after the breasts, legs and wings are removed from the bird, the carcasses are forced through a sieve under high pressure to separate bone from the edible tissue. This paste-like poultry product is then, like the beef above, treated with a small amount of ammonium hydroxide as an anti-microbial agent. The definition of 'edible tissue' here could be considered a stretch by many, essentially referring to anything left on the bones, including nerves, blood vessels, cartilage and skin, as well as the miniscule amount of actual meat. The resulting product is essentially the poultry equivalent of 'pink slime' above . . . 'white slime' if you would. Mechanically separated poultry is allowed to be sold in the EU. Hurrah! Mechanically separated beef used to be a thing as well, but fear of mad cow disease or Bovine spongiform encephalopathy, which can be transmitted through consumption of the brain and nervous system of infected cattle, put a stop to the practice of forcing cow vertebrae, complete with spinal cord, through a sieve.

Enfin, we have the *pièce de résistance* of processed meat, the wonderfully visceral sounding 'meat slurry' . . . mmmm. Meat slurry or emulsified meat is, quite literally, a liquefied meat product. Meat, most commonly chicken (although beef and pork can also be processed as such), is first finely ground and mixed with water. This mush is treated with either an emulsifier or placed in a centrifuge to separate the fat from the muscle. The resulting liquefied protein is then frozen. This is the most likely provenance of the contents found in cheaper 'chicken nuggets' or other shaped chicken products, for instance.

To be clear, all of these reconstituted products are 100 per cent from beef or chicken or turkey or pork (they may not entirely be muscular in origin, and come with added water and a spritz of ammonium hydroxide), and are perfectly safe to eat, even if their highly industrialised methods of production are unpleasant sounding and off-putting to many, vegetarian or not.

So, why could the consumption of ultra-processed foods be linked to weight gain? First of all, given what the chicken meat (or perhaps more accurately protein of chicken origin) has been through before ending up on your plate – sieved, emulsified, cen-trifuged and lord knows what else – there is going to be little in the way of flavour remaining. So you have to ADD flavour to the white slime or meat slurry, which will come from salt, sugar, fat and flavour enhancers. Sure, there are often other spices added as well, but let's face it, we are not in the middle of an obesity crisis because we've had a bit too much cumin or paprika. Even then you are still looking at a flavoured liquefied chicken paste, so you have to add stabilisers and starch and whatever else to hold it all together. Then you obviously have to batter and fry it, before the modern wonder of a chicken nugget is served to you with a side of BBQ sauce and fries.

That is the problem with many (but not all) ultra-processed foods; because the processing strips out much of the flavour, which has to be replaced to be made palatable, you often end up consuming more sugar, salt and fat as a result. Most of us, unless we peer at the back of the packaging from which our frozen fish fingers have emerged (honestly, ask yourself when was the last time you did that?), certainly have no idea at all how much salt, sugar and fat has been added. In addition, when plant-based prod-ucts undergo ultra-processing, they often lose more than just their flavour (which is replaced), but much of their fibre as well (which is often not replaced). So on average (and it is an average and not an absolute rule), ultra-processed foods are typically higher in salt, sugar and fat, and lower in fibre, which is what makes that lovely 'protein of chicken origin' nugget oh so moreish, and also oh so very calorically available. It is easy to eat and even easier to extract the calories. Compare that to eating a piece of chicken breast, even if it has been battered and fried, where you can control the amount of seasoning and fat that goes in.

So what does this have to do with calories?

ULTRA-PROCESSED FOODS RESULT IN LESS DIET-INDUCED THERMOGENESIS

The equation of caloric availability includes not only the amount of energy it takes to digest and metabolise the food in question, but crucially, how much heat is given off in the process, so-called diet-induced thermogenesis. There was a study, conducted by Sadie Barr and Jonathan Wright from Pomona College, Claremont, California, published in 2010, that explored whether the degree to which a food had been processed influenced diet-induced thermogenesis.[10] Since the publication of this study was just a year after Monteiro proposed the concept of ultra-processed food, the term had yet to enter the diet-and-nutrition vernacular and was not used by Barr and Wright.

Barr and Wright recruited seventeen lean and healthy volunteers (twelve women and five men), and got them each to consume two different meals, one labelled 'wholefood' and one labelled 'processed food', on two different days. Both meals were simple cheese sandwiches. The 'wholefood' sandwich was comprised of multi-grain bread (containing whole sunflower seeds and other whole-grain kernels) and cheddar cheese, while the 'processed' sandwich was made of white bread and a processed cheese product. Given that this was a clinical study, the bread used, multi-grain or white, would have been of the supermarket, mass-produced variety, and would have been classed as ultra-processed by NOVA. The Cheddar cheese used would have been a Group 3 processed product, and the processed cheese product would have been ultra-processed. But as I've said, there is a whole spectrum of ultra-processed food. The two different meals were matched and consisted of 600-calorie (2,520kJ, one and a half sandwiches) or 800-calorie portions (3,360kJ, two sandwiches), with 60 per cent of the energy for each meal coming from the bread, and the remaining 40 per

cent from the cheese. Each subject was asked to choose a preferred portion size and consumed this portion size for both meals,
with the order in which they were eaten, wholefood or processed
food first, randomly chosen. Subjects were asked to fast for twelve
hours prior to the beginning of each trial meal, and not to partici-
pate in any strenuous exercise during the day of the trial. To provide a baseline, basal metabolic rate (BMR) was measured before
the meal. Subjects then had twenty minutes to eat and were asked
to return for six metabolic rate measurements at hourly intervals.

What were the results? Well, on average, diet-induced thermogenesis after eating the wholefood sandwiches was 137 calories,
or 20 per cent of the energy of the meal, which was nearly double
that of the processed sandwiches, at 73 calories, or 10.7 per cent
of the energy of the meal! That means that even though the sandwiches contained *exactly the same number of calories*, the body
has to spend nearly twice the number of calories to metabolise the
wholefood sandwich compared to the processed sandwich. Put
another way, eating the processed sandwich means you absorb 10
per cent more calories than if you had eaten the wholefood sandwich! The strength of this study was that because each subject ate
both meals in random order, they were their own experimental
control. There was no concern about genetics or body size or sex.
The weakness of this study was that it was small, encompassed
only two meals, and, crucially, only examined cheese sandwiches.
But it was an important first experiment.

So the question of course is why there was this difference in
diet-induced thermogenesis. Now, Barr and Wright had tried
their best to match the sandwiches for nutritional profile, but for
this particular study, decided that they had to match the calories
as a priority. This meant that there were then differences in the
macronutrient composition of the sandwiches. The wholefood
sandwich was 40 per cent carbohydrate, 39 per cent fat, and 20
per cent protein; whereas the processed sandwich was 50 per cent

carbohydrate, 33 per cent fat, and 15 per cent protein. The whole-food sandwiches had 10 per cent less carbs and 5 per cent more protein, and crucially, three times the amount of dietary fibre than the processed sandwiches. It was the higher-protein and fibre content that decreased the caloric availability of the wholefood sandwich, and likely correspondingly increased the amount of energy it took to digest and metabolise it.

ULTRA-PROCESSED DIETS CAUSE YOU TO EAT MORE

Now, if it wasn't bad enough that ultra-processed diets are more calorically available, evidence is emerging that they also make you eat more! In a study performed in 2019 by Kevin Hall and colleagues from the US National Institute of Health in Bethesda, Maryland, ten male and ten female healthy and weight-stable adults were recruited to a twenty-eight-day in-house study (a pretty long time to be staying at a clinical research unit!).[11] Subjects were randomly assigned to either an ultra-processed or unprocessed diet (following the NOVA taxonomy) for two weeks, followed immediately by the alternate diet for the final two weeks. During each diet phase, the subjects were presented with three daily meals and could eat as much or as little as they wanted. (Hey! How come I never get recruited to eat-as-much-as-you-like studies?) The meals were designed to be as well matched as possible across diets for total calories, energy density, macronutrients, fibre, sugar and salt. However, the ultra-processed versus unprocessed meals differed substantially in the proportion of added total sugar (54 per cent versus 1 per cent, respectively), insoluble to total fibre (77 per cent versus 16 per cent, respectively) and saturated to total fat (34 per cent versus 19 per cent).

What were the results? Keeping in mind that the subjects were not limited in the amount of food they could eat, they ate on average 500 more calories a day when on the ultra-processed diet compared to being on the unprocessed diet. Five hundred calories! Neither the order of the diet assignment, nor sex, nor starting BMI had significant effects on the difference in food intake between the diets. Unsurprisingly, participants gained, on average, 1 kilogram during the ultra-processed diet and lost the same amount of weight during the unprocessed diet. Remember that each dietary phase only lasted two weeks.

There are some particularly interesting things to note about this experiment.

First, those extra 500 calories per day that were being consumed during the ultra-processed phase? They came from 280 calories in extra carbs and 230 calories in extra fat, but the amount of protein that was consumed stayed nearly constant. In 2005, writing in the journal *Obesity Reviews*, Australian scientists Stephen J. Simpson and David Raubenheimer from the University of Sydney proposed 'the protein leverage hypothesis' as a possible driver of the obesity epidemic.[12] They argued that a major driving force in what and how much we eat is to maintain a certain level of protein in our diet, which across a number of very different species, from flies to mice to humans, is around 15 per cent. If a diet contains comparatively less protein, but more fat and carbs, then one will eat more total calories in order to maintain the 15 per cent of protein, because this is what is required for the healthy maintenance of our bodies. The inverse was also demonstrated to be true; that is, if a diet contained comparatively more protein, then less fat and carbs, and hence fewer total calories, were consumed. The remarkable stability of absolute protein intake between the ultra-processed versus the unprocessed diet (14 per cent versus 15.6 per cent of calories, respectively), supports the protein leverage hypothesis. It suggests that because the ultra-processed diet contained proportionally less protein, the subjects in the experiment had to increase their total food intake by 500 calories a day in an attempt to maintain a constant protein intake.

Second, the total amount of fibre consumed by subjects in this experiment was remarkably similar between the ultra-processed and unprocessed diets. This surprised me because, as discussed, ultra-processed food is not renowned for its rich fibre content. However, upon closer reading of the paper, buried in the text was the statement that in order to achieve fibre parity, beverages with dissolved fibre supplements were included in the ultra-processed meals, precisely because they were so low in fibre. What this meant was that 77 per cent of the fibre present in the unprocessed meals was insoluble, compared to 16 per cent of the fibre in the ultra-processed meals, with the rest composed of soluble fibre. Insoluble fibre is almost completely unavailable to humans. It goes right through us, and we poop it out. Our microbiome, however, is able to ferment a significant percentage of soluble fibre into short-chain fatty acids that we can use as fuel, allowing us to extract much of the calories from soluble fibre. Thus, ultra-processed diets are more calorically available not only because they have proportionally less protein and more carbs and fat, but also because they have far less fibre, of which a higher proportion is soluble.

Third, Hall and colleagues also measured diet-induced thermogenesis during the experiment, but in contrast to Barr and Wright's cheese sandwich experiment, found no measurable differences in post-meal energy expenditure between the ultra-processed and unprocessed diets. So how come a group does one experiment that reveals one result, and another group does a similar experiment and shows a different result? Was someone lying? Was someone wrong? Hold your horses, everyone; this is how science works. For one thing, although the experiments were similar, there were some important differences. Barr and Wright's study only took measurements for two meals, each comprising only one item of food; in contrast, Hall and colleagues were examining subjects undergoing a far longer-term experiment, and consuming two entirely different diets. The truth is, these are only the opening salvos to an important aspect of dietary and nutritional science. More experiments are going to need to be performed, with more participants and in a broad range of conditions, before we can say anything conclusive about the impact of ultra-processed foods on diet-induced thermogenesis.

Finally, using the cost of ingredients obtained from a local branch of a large supermarket chain, the authors of the study estimated that the weekly cost for ingredients to prepare 2000kcal per day of ultra-processed meals was, in US dollars, $106 versus $151 for the unprocessed meals. The ultra-processed meals were almost a third cheaper, which has implications for the affordability of trying to eat healthily, particularly for the less privileged in society. I will return to this theme in the next chapter, where I shall explore the relationship between privilege and calories.

HUMANS ARE A TERRIBLE JUDGE OF CALORIE CONTENT IN FOODS THAT CONTAIN FAT AND CARBS

One other intriguing concept that has emerged over the past few years is the possibility that we are hard-wired in our response to certain characteristics of ultra-processed foods; specifically, our response to the combination of fat and carbs that are typically present. Now clearly there are non-processed foods that contain fat and carbs together – roast potatoes (once again, in goose fat) and anything battered and fried come to mind, along with butter on homemade bread, butter on boiled new potatoes, in fact, butter on anything! – but these clearly are not going to sit in the 'healthy' category. However, many ultra-processed foods have that magic combination of being high in fat and carbs, while simultaneously being low in protein and fibre.

An experiment conducted by a colleague of mine, Dana Small from Yale University, in 2018, explored the way we simple humans respond to foods high in fat, foods high in carbs, and foods high in both fat and carbs.[13] Small employed an eBay-style auction paradigm to assess how much someone values a specific food item, coupled with using magnetic resonance imaging or MRI to scan the subject's brain in order to see which part of the brain is activated during the process. What Small did was to create a set of pictures of snacks falling into one of three categories: those with most of their calories coming from fat, from carbohydrate, or from fat and carbohydrates. All participants first rated these snacks for liking and familiarity (no sense in including pictures of Jammie Dodgers or chocolate Hobnobs, for instance, if the participant detests them or doesn't know of their existence), estimated energy density and caloric content. They were then given €5 (Euros) and told they could bid between €0 and €5 against the computer to purchase snacks depicted in the pictures. They were told that one item would be selected at random, and if the participant's bid was higher than the computer's, he or she was then able to purchase the item and receive the remainder of the €5 in cash. Otherwise, the participant received the entire €5 but did not get the item. The participant's brain was scanned throughout the duration of this experiment. The study was designed so that under these circumstances, the optimum strategy would be to bid what one believes is the value of the item. This type of auction paradigm, engaging in the act of bidding against someone (or in this instance against a computer) has been shown to be a better way of uncovering someone's true perception of value, compared to simply asking, 'Hey, how much do you think this is worth?'.

So how about those scores on the door? Interestingly, participants were far better at estimating the calorie content of fat snacks compared to the carbohydrate snacks, and were absolutely hopeless in trying to guess how many calories were present in fat-and-carbohydrate snacks. In addition, participants were willing to pay significantly more for foods with fat and carbohydrate compared to fat or carbohydrate foods; greater than would be expected from adding together the bids for just fat and just carbohydrate foods. And similarly, while the area of the brain that encodes reward (the oooooooh feeling when you see or eat a chocolate cake, for instance) was activated by most of the images, it lights up like a Christmas tree with images of fat-and-carbohydrate foods, the response far greater than the individual responses from fat foods and carbohydrate foods.

What this experiment demonstrated was that we simple humans are awful at judging the amount of calories in foods high in both fat and carbs. To make things worse, we find these fat-and-carbs foods to be more rewarding, calorie for calorie, than those containing only fat or only carbohydrate, and it is largely down to the way our brains are wired. So not only do we love that hedonistic mixture of fat and carbs, most of the time we don't even know how much of it we're eating! It is double jeopardy. If you think about it, foods in nature that are naturally high in both fat and carbs (as opposed to something like French fries that are high in carbs and cooked in fat) are actually extremely rare. Foods high in carbs would include most root vegetables, fruit, honey and grains, but all are almost fat free. High in fat? Animal-based foods mostly, but these would be very low in carbs. Coconuts and avocados are high in fat and naturally sweet, I guess, but they are hardly sugary, and their availability is (or at least used to be) geographically restricted. In fact, the one example of a food that is naturally high in both fat and carbs is actually ubiquitously abundant and is the food that all mammals begin their life with: milk.

Milk is a food designed to be easy to consume (it is a liquid) and to be very calorically dense because the priority of any baby mammal is to grow as quickly as possible to reduce their chances of becoming tiger food (unless you are a baby tiger of course). It is also one of the only times (if not the only time, but I always find it wise to hedge, because absolutes have a way of coming back to bite you in the backside) that we end up drinking our calories. We eat fruit, with juice being a modern phenomenon; and honey is a liquid of course, but you don't eat a great deal of it at any time and I don't think it is a major source of calories for humans. One could speculate (and it can really only be speculation) that our innate attraction to foods high in both fat and carbs is a primal response, hard-wired into us as mammals so we instinctively seek out our mother's teat at the first opportunity and consume as much as possible as quickly as possible. Regardless of the attractive evo-lutionary story, there does appear to be a biologically plausible mechanism to explain why our response, as humans, is to overeat in this contemporary environment rich in ultra-processed foods that are high in fat and carbs.

PLANT-BASED 'DAIRY'

Because milk is pasteurised, certainly the stuff you buy in the shops, it is considered a minimally processed food; Group 1 in the NOVA classification. Which brings us back to where we start-ed this chapter. One of the fastest-growing areas in food at the moment is plant-based dairy alternatives. The rapidly expanding vegan market has clearly played a significant role in this; but many who are not vegan also embrace these plant-based alternatives be-cause they are perceived to be healthier for you. Plant-based milk, for instance, now represents 15 per cent of the total milk market. Think about that for a second, 15 per cent of the milk market is not actually milk at all!

I am ethnically Chinese, so have drunk soy milk all my life, although we never actually called it 'milk'. Rather we called it 豆浆 (doujiang), which literally translates to 'soybean broth'. This was originally a by-product of the tofu-manufacturing process and it is typically drunk slightly sweetened, either warm or cold. Chinese people, certainly when I was younger, would have never countenanced using soy milk as a dairy alternative, putting it, for example, into coffee or tea or on cereal . . . but you white people gotta do what you gotta do. Given that the original soy milk was a direct side product of making tofu, which has similarities to how cheese is made, where the protein solids are curdled out of solution, I am guessing the original soy broth of my youth would be a NOVA classified Group 3 food. It was only a fairly recent thing, certainly within the twenty-first century, that industrial manufacturing magic was used to thicken it slightly, giving it a 'fattier' taste to more closely resemble cows' milk so that you could use it in coffee or cereal. If we compare the amount of protein found in soy milk, at 3.3 grams per 100 millilitres, to that of cows' milk, at 3.6 grams per 100 millilitres, they are almost identical. However, to this day, the 'soy milk' available in coffee shops and supermarkets the world over still tastes weird to me . . . it is recognisable in taste as the 'soybean broth' from my youth, but it is slightly too sweet for my liking, and leaves a weird sensation on my palate.

Almonds and coconuts are both naturally high in fat, so their resulting 'milks' have that 'fatty' consistency, even though they clearly taste entirely different. It is personal taste, of course, but while I enjoy coconut flavour, I prefer it in a Thai curry or perhaps a pina colada (but not getting caught in the rain), not in my coffee and almost certainly not in my tea (ick)! And don't even think about getting Jane started on what she thinks about coconut milk in tea . . .

Another major product available is 'oat milk'. Now, until I looked into it, it was entirely a mystery to me how, given the source material, you could turn oats into anything resembling milk. As it turns out, oat milk is 10 per cent oats, which have been soaked, giving the required white colour. The fatty taste and consistency comes from rapeseed oil and other emulsifiers (yum!), and it is then fortified with a whole heap of vitamins and minerals so that you get any significant nutritional value from drinking it at all. This and the closely related 'quinoa milk' are clearly only possible because of high-tech industrialised processes.

Other products within this category are plant-based cheeses, butter, yogurts, crème fraîche and ice-creams. Take vegan 'cheese' for instance; many of the fancier pizza parlours here in the UK now provide a vegan-cheese option. In fact, at time of writing, the UK now has its first and only 'plant-based cheesemonger'. Opened in 2019 by sisters Charlotte and Rachel Stevens in Brixton Village, south London, La Fauxmagerie has been doing a roaring trade. They have, however, incurred the wrath of Dairy UK, who asked La Fauxmagerie to stop calling its produce 'cheese'.[14] They say that using the word 'cheese' for anything other than real dairy products is misleading, because plant-based alternatives do not have the same nutritional content. The shop owners have fired back, saying they are clearly labelling their food. I have to say that I am on the side of the Stevens sisters here. While I understand that vegan 'cheese' is clearly not cheese, they only sell vegan products in their store. I mean, the name of their store is literally 'Faux'-magerie, so how can you accuse them of misleading anyone or mis-selling anything? Will there come a time where vegan 'cheese' makes that same leap into the mainstream? Undoubtedly. This seems, however, a little way away yet, because all of the vegan cheese I tasted, even in those fancy pizza joints, still tasted plasticky to me.

Aside from the original soy broth of my youth and coconut milk, all of the other plant-based dairy products, including the modern version of soy milk, are classed as ultra-processed products. Yet – and I don't want to generalise, but I will – the #fitspo influencer uploading an image of their breakfast of almond-milk and steel-cut oats with a scatter of blueberries onto Instagram is not, in a million years, going to be caught dead with a chicken nugget. Even if they did surreptitiously sneak a dirty burger or hotdog every now and then, they certainly wouldn't be posting or blogging about it. Yet both are ultra-processed products containing many more than five ingredients, mostly unpronounceable chemical names, that your grandparents would most certainly not have recognised as food. These are some of the other characteristics of ultra-processed foods. And just as an aside, what is this magic thing about five ingredients or less anyway? Why is that automatically better? If I use Chinese five-spice powder in a recipe, that would presumably count as one of the five ingredients. However, what if I added in the typical components of five-spice powder, so star anise, fennel seeds, Szechuan peppercorns, cloves and cinnamon, separately into a dish? Does that suddenly mean my dish becomes 'false' or 'dirty'? Just asking for a friend.

VEGAN 'MEAT', BEYOND THE IMPOSSIBLE

Most manufacturers of food, industrially processed or not, vegan or not, typically try to market their products as if they are nature's own or mum's home cookin' or both, for good reason. It gives the consumer that warm fuzzy feeling of childhood as they are consuming their microwaved vegan chilli burrito. Two notable exceptions, however, are Beyond Meat and Impossible Foods, who are both food companies in a nakedly high-tech ultra-processed battle to fool the consumer's eyes, nose and taste-buds with 'fake meat'. These are very different beasts from the protein-less vegan pulled pork, where flavoured jackfruit replaces the pork with little to no processing. In developing the 'Beyond' and 'Impossible' burgers, both manufacturers are trying to make these vegan burgers taste, feel and even cook like meat. They are not trying to make vegan food palatable to omnivores, they are trying to make a plant-based burger where not even committed carnivores can tell they are not eating meat.

Just observe the use of language by the founder of Beyond Meat, Ethan Brown, in an interview for the *San Francisco Chronicle*[15]:

'The texture of meat is complex, and there's a beauty to how unique it is.'

The innovation of Beyond Burger is in using biomedical equipment to rethink how a base of pea protein, with mung-bean protein and coconut fat added for textural variety, are dispersed throughout the patty.

'How do we increase the heterogeneity of a bite so you're getting the nuances of tendons and fat, fat bursting, different cuts of protein, bits of gristle?'

Is it wrong that my mouth just started watering?

Anyway, if you think that sounds visceral, Impossible Foods has gone one step 'beyond' (boom boom . . . I'm here all week, folks), and developed a plant-based burger that bleeds! Do they use beetroot juice? Wine? Nope, although, come to think of it, a wine-burger has certain appeal. They actually use the molecule that gives blood its red colour, heme, which is iron rich and responsible for the oxygen-carrying capacity of blood, except of course it is a plant-based heme, found in the roots of soy plants. It gives Impossible Burger its meat-like flavour and ability to morph from pink to brown as it cooks, so you could choose to have it medium-rare, for instance. So while Beyond Burgers are pre-flavoured to taste and feel like cooked meat, Impossible Burgers are designed to create meat flavour upon cooking. In order to generate enough heme for all the burgers they want to sell, Impossible Foods have not set-up a giant soy-plant root-juicing facility; rather, they have genetically engineered yeast cells in enormous vats to produce prodigious amounts of blood-red, iron-y heme. Nakedly high-tech ultra-processed, as I said.

The founder of Impossible Foods, ex-Stanford professor Pat Brown, is entirely open about his goals. In a piece he wrote for the website *Medium*, he says:

'*Our first product, the Impossible Burger, uses 75 per cent less water, generates 87 per cent less greenhouse gases, requires 95 per cent less land and 100 per cent fewer cows ... If everyone who eats beef burgers today chose Impossible Burgers instead, the positive impact on our planet and global health would be profound.*'[16]

Both Browns (Ethan and Pat) are unrelated, both are in fierce competition, but both are also united in their aim to change the world. Their intended audience isn't the hipster, the organic-minded or even the vegetarian. They are trying to replace meat entirely, without the consumers being able to tell the difference. Given their high-tech DNA, both California-based companies are more akin to Silicon Valley start-ups than traditional food manufacturers, and both have managed to attract hundreds of millions of dollars in investment. The Bill and Melinda Gates foundation, for instance, are famous backers of Beyond Meat, while Impossible Foods have attracted backing from celebrities such as musicians Jay-Z and Will.i.am, and institutional backing from Google. As a result, Beyond Burgers are actually stocked in the fresh meat fridges of some of the major American supermarket chains, while restaurants across the USA are selling Impossible Burgers.[17] In fact, the big beasts are now getting involved, with Burger King rolling out 'Impossible' Whoppers throughout the USA and in a limited number of their international outlets, including here in the UK. There was even an outlet in Brooklyn, New York that got into trouble because they were selling actual moo-moo-based whoppers as 'Impossible' ones![18]

Will they be successful? OK, they are already successful, but will they change the world? I guess only time will tell. I have tried a Beyond Burger at an establishment here in Cambridge and while it is not quite a beef burger (yet), it is getting pretty darn close.

It is definitely a far cry from those frozen Quorn patties that simply get drier and drier as you cook them, till you get some mushroom-flavoured disk; tasty to be sure, but still a dried-up mushroom-flavoured disk!

ARE ULTRA-PROCESSED FOODS BY DEFINITION BAD?

Monteiro wrote in a 2017 commentary for the journal *Public Health Nutrition*:

'*The evidence so far shows that displacement of minimally processed foods and freshly prepared dishes and meals by ultra-processed products is associated with unhealthy dietary nutrient profiles and several diet-related non-communicable diseases.*'[19]

This statement is undoubtedly true for many ultra-processed foods. However, because the term covers such a broad spectrum of different foods, from otherwise minimally processed foods with a few industrial additives, to those that have been almost completely reconstructed from their base constituents, it is not going to be true for all ultra-processed foods. I guess that is my issue with the concept of 'ultra-processed'. While as a definition – encompassing foods that have been industrially processed in a way that is difficult or impossible to replicate in a domestic setting – it is clear enough it is, however, ill-suited as an arbiter of how healthy or unhealthy a particular food might be.

To be crystal clear, I am not denying that we need to limit consumption of foods that are high in fat, sugar and/or salt, while simultaneously being low in protein or fibre or both. We are, as a society, undoubtedly consuming too much of such foods. It's just that 'ultra-processed' includes many foods that are neither. Take the oft-maligned humble meal of hamburger and fries. Yes, there are burgers of the frozen variety that have added lean finely textured beef and fries that are constructed from reconstituted potatoes, and both are likely to be high in sugar, salt and fat. But you could also have a burger made from minced beef with less than 15 per cent fat and just a bit of salt and pepper, together with potatoes that have been hand cut, and oven baked in olive oil, which coincidentally is what I'm having for dinner tonight. You can have a battered and fried chicken nugget made with either meat-slurry or a piece of chicken breast. You can have a fish goujon or a fish finger.

Monteiro then goes on to say:

'Ultra-processed products are also troublesome from social, cultural, economic, political and environmental points of view. We conclude that the ever-increasing production and consumption of these products is a world crisis, to be confronted, checked and reversed . . .'[20]

These are bold statements. I agree that because many of the ultra-processed foods of the high in sugar/fat/salt/low-protein/low-fibre variety are cheap to produce, and because of their long shelf-lives are easy to store and transport, they are inexpensive and more likely to be purchased and consumed by those less privileged in society (this is a major theme that I will explore in the next chapter). I also agree that the wholesale exportation of our Western 'fast-food' brands threatens to overwhelm local cuisine. The ubiquity with which these foods are available does require a sober and non-hysterical debate.

But at the same time it is intriguing, to me at least, that other ultra-processed foods have not only avoided being tarred by the same brush, but instead somehow managed to successfully virtue-signal a halo of health. I have discussed the panoply of plant-based dairy replacements and faux-meat burgers, but many other 'premium' ultra-processed foods are available that find their way into higher-end supermarkets and restaurants. From a processing standpoint, there is really no difference between oat-milk crème fraîche and ice-cream, or a frozen burger patty with added 'pink slime' and a burger made from soy protein that bleeds heme sourced from genetically engineered yeast. From a nutritional perspective, aside from the obvious difference in the presence of animal-based saturated fat in the ice-cream and the burger, oat-milk has a lot of oil and emulsifiers and other additives, and a faux-meat burger is still high in sugar, salt and fat; looking through a different lens, one might even consider them a 'junk food'!

I am an unashamed champion of improving our diets in order to try and stem the current tsunami of diet-related illnesses, and there are countless foods, many that have been referred to in this chapter, that we undoubtedly have to eat a lot less of. However, I fear that the ultra-processed concept is too blunt a tool, and, even worse, that it is currently being used as another cudgel to food-shame others, while at the same time, the privileged in society celebrate and congratulate themselves for eating similarly processed foods that simply have better PR.

CHAPTER 8

Privilege and calories

I love my food. I love the planning of the dishes, the sourcing of the ingredients, the preparation, the cooking, and of course the *raison d'être* and climax to the whole affair, I love eating the food and particularly sharing it with others. In fact, the only bit of the whole process I'm not so keen on is the washing up after.

Not surprising then that my key domestic responsibility is putting food on to the table. I cook every evening, except on Fridays when we get a curry or Chinese takeaway. Typically, the weekday meals, because of the pesky inconvenience of having to be at work during the day, are more simple affairs. Stir-fries feature, either with chicken, or on my 'vegan evenings' tofu, served with steamed rice, of course. Asian-style soup and noodles are a go-to easy meal, as long as the all-important stock, always coming from the bones or carcass of some weekend roast dinner, is already made. Quick pasta dishes, such as my tagliatelle with creamy bacon and porcini sauce, and any kind of marinated (always for an hour at least, overnight if possible) grilled meat or fish, in the oven or on the hob top in the winter and on the BBQ when the weather is nice, served with either steamed veg or salad, and rice, couscous or potatoes, with a killer sauce (you always need a killer sauce).

Weekends, however, provide the luxury of time, and along with it the preparation of dishes that cannot be rushed. Saturdays mean casseroles and stews in the winter, these include British classics such as beef or lamb stew with dumplings, or my ragu, made with pancetta, minced beef, minced pork and (the secret ingredient) chopped chicken livers, cooked in a tomato sauce low and slow in the oven for three to four hours and served with spaghetti or layered in a lasagne. There is also the opportunity to cook cheaper cuts of meat such as brisket. My favourite brisket dish is 'Chinese black beef'. The joint of beef is braised in stock with dark soy sauce, Chinese Shaoxing rice wine and an absolute ton of garlic, like nearly forty cloves. It sounds like a scary amount of garlic, but once you've coloured it a little in hot oil to burn off the harshest of the volatiles and braised it for three to four hours, and then mushed it all up, it actually thickens the sauce and you end up with a deep sweet umami flavour. Slice and serve it up with some veg of your choice, steamed rice and an ice-cold beer . . . oh my word, it is heaven.

Sundays bring the joy of a roast dinner. Chicken, pork or lamb mostly. If cooking a leg of lamb or pork, then I roast it at a higher temperature for a shorter period of time, if it is the shoulder, because of the higher fat content, then low and slow. On special occasions, I splash out and get a rib of beef. Always served with roast potatoes and a killer gravy (oooh yeah). Once every few weeks I mix it up and cook a family favourite, Hainanese chicken rice. My maternal grandfather is from the island of Hainan in the South China Sea, and the version of the dish that I cook has been handed down from my grandfather, to my mother and then to me. Chicken rice was originally a peasant dish. It is, in effect, poached chicken, with the poaching liquor used to make the rice (hence chicken rice), a soup, the sauce and the fiery ginger, chilli and garlic dip. In days gone by, one modest-sized chicken would have fed quite a big family, with just a little portion of meat each. But yet, because all of the accompaniments were made with the cooking stock, the flavour of the chicken was infused throughout the entire meal. Today, of course, the chicken-to-accompaniment ratio has shifted, and we have all the chicken that we need (and more).

So in normal times, that is kind of the cooking schedule that I would keep. However, March to July 2020, when I wrote much of this book, including this chapter, was not a normal time. In the UK, as was true for the majority of other countries in the world, most of us were locked down in our homes because of the Covid-19 pandemic. That meant working from home and interminable Zoom meetings. However, it also meant time for weekend-style cooking every day of the week! I would, on a Monday, be able to put some beef short-ribs or pork loin-ribs into a marinade in the morning, pop them in the oven in the afternoon, and low and slow them to perfection just in time for dinner. I could, on a Wednesday, have crispy aromatic duck, generously dusted with Chinese five spice powder, slow roasted and served with rice pancakes, together with my 'black eggs' – hard-boiled duck eggs steeped in a gingery sweet dark soy and five-spice sauce. To supply my habit, I found a very good butcher online that sold ethically reared meat and delivered direct to my front door within forty-eight hours.

We (well, Jane) even succumbed to the embarrassingly middle-class lockdown cliché of tending to a sourdough starter. This aspect had, shall we say, mixed results. Jane managed to use the starter (that constantly needed feeding; they say it is like owning a pet, and they, whoever 'they' are, were correct!) to create wonderfully poufy sourdough cinnamon rolls topped with a cream cheese icing. We certainly ate way too many of those. Actually making sourdough bread, however, that was less successful. The very first leavened or raised (as opposed to flat) bread was, in all likelihood, a sourdough, given that it only required flour, some yeast that had stowed away on the grains, and water. Someone, thousands of years ago, probably left out some gruel by mistake, and came back to a bubbling concoction that when mixed with more flour and baked, suddenly resembled what we now recognise as bread. After multiple attempts at stretching and folding, trying both overnight proving in the fridge and proving at room temperature for a few hours, baking in an oven with a tray of boiling water as well as trying out baking in a casserole, and eventually resorting to trying to 'science' our way through this procedure with thermometers and measuring humidity, we have ended up with something edible but still incredibly dense. Who knew it would be quite so complicated?

But the truth of the matter was, it was a first-world distraction . . . entertainment even. Jane and I were both fully paid and managed to work effectively from home during the lockdown. We had plenty of high-quality food, probably too much, that we were able to prepare in a multitude of delicious ways. We had a garden and could enjoy the sun, and the only thing we had to worry about were our expanding waistlines, which we tried valiantly to mitigate by getting regular exercise. We were undeniably comfortable during lockdown and, as it dragged on into the second and third months, became acutely aware of our privilege.

Many many millions, in the UK alone, were not as fortunate.

FOOD INSECURITY

This will be surprising to many people, but the UK, in spite being the sixth wealthiest country in the world, suffers from a unconscionably high level of food insecurity. Say it ain't so . . . I hear a chorus of fellow middle-class people ask. I don't see starving children in the streets. We're not in the middle of a famine or war.

Here's the thing: what we are talking about is not starvation, which ostensibly occurs because of famine and war. In truth, there is absolutely no excuse today for anyone to starve, and when it happens, it is mostly for the worst reasons of all: political inertia and inexpediency in the international community. Food insecurity is different from starvation and is defined as a 'limited access to food due to lack of money or other resources'. It may be less acute but is actually more insidious because it is able to hide in plain sight, certainly from those of us living in our food-secure bubble. According to the Food and Agriculture Organisation (FAO) of the United Nations, the level of food insecurity can be measured on the Food Insecurity and Experience Scale,[1] shown in the figure below. It ranges from 'mild' food insecurity, which is when someone worries about their ability to obtain food, to 'moderate', which can be having to compromise on the quality and variety of food, or even reducing quantities and skipping meals, to 'severe', which means experiencing consistent hunger. When was the last time most of you reading this book even had to worry about your ability to obtain food? Probably the same as me; that is, never. And no, drinking all your money away while being a student at university and having to eat a tin of beans for dinner does not count.

Mild food insecurity	Moderate food insecurity		Severe food insecurity
Worrying about ability to obtain food	Compromising quality and variety of food	Reducing quantities, skipping meals	Experiencing hunger

In June 2017, UNICEF (The United Nations Children's Fund) reported that in the UK, 1 in 5 children under age fifteen lived with an adult who was moderately or severely food insecure, of which half were severely food insecure. That is 2.2 million severely food insecure people, making the UK one of, if not the, worst-performing nations in the EU.[2] In the US, 11.1 per cent, or around 14.3 million, of households were food insecure at some time during 2018, with 4.3 per cent (5.6 million) of households being severely food insecure.[3] This means that in 2018, 37.2 million people in the world's wealthiest country lived in food-insecure households.

The problem is that the 'average' situation in many wealthy countries, like the UK and US, hides huge variations in food security, which are tightly linked to socioeconomic status. Thus we are faced with two juxtaposed challenges: high levels of household food insecurity and yet a growing global pandemic, this time non-communicable, of obesity and diet-related disease. Both challenges are underpinned by an unequal food system, in which some of us are happily sourcing ethically reared meat and 'struggling' with sourdough, while many others are actually struggling to provide healthy, sustainable and diverse diets for themselves and their family.

Consider that in 'normal' pre-pandemic times, there were 1.3 million kids on free school meals in the UK, and for the majority of these children, what they eat at school represents the majority of their daily calories. This has resulted in the phenomenon of holiday hunger, where these children are simply not getting enough (or the right) food when the schools are shut. Think about it, these are kids, from underprivileged households, whose parents mostly have jobs, yet need help to pay for their meals. In a survey of more than four hundred UK schools in 2019, the Association of School and College Leaders found 43 per cent of schools were offering families help with food.[4] These included a few schools that were running actual food banks (!!), but most involved schools providing food parcels on a more occasional basis. I'm sorry, but I refuse to consider this 'normal' in any way. How is there not more uproar about the fact that this is still happening in a rich country in the twenty-first century?

What the Covid-19 pandemic lockdown did was to make things worse for the poorest in society, laying bare these inequalities and forcing us all to stick our heads out of the bubble to look about. Some of us remained fully employed, continuing to work remotely, on Zoom and Teams and whatnot; other employees of businesses big and small were furloughed, in the UK at least; the professional freelancers, filmmakers, cameramen and soundwomen (and vice versa), musicians and others, were not so lucky, but the many that I know, somehow managed; and business and restaurant owners, I salute you. But then there were the many millions, those who could least afford to, that simply lost their job, with no safety net whatsoever. And with every school in the UK shuttered, the government had to come up with a voucher scheme to try and help feed those who had relied on schools for their meals. More than two hundred thousand kids fell through the net, receiving no support at all, and ending up going hungry.[5] It was a tragedy. Criminal, even.

So why and how does food insecurity link to obesity and other diet-related disease?

BODYWEIGHT IS NOT A CHOICE

I mentioned at the beginning of Chapter 5 that my research focuses on the genetics of obesity.

OK, stop, I can hear the questions from sceptics in the peanut gallery already. How can obesity be blamed on genes? People were not fat thirty to forty years ago, whereas they are now. How do you explain that? Surely people are simply eating too much rubbish?

I facetiously called out the peanut-eating sceptics, but actually, these are perfectly valid questions, that most people in society would ask. So let us acknowledge a few irrefutable facts. First, it is true that the ONLY way that one can gain weight is to eat more calories than you burn, it is physics after all; second, it is true that the prevalence of those living with obesity has rapidly risen over the past thirty years; third, it is true that obesity is a serious public health problem.

Aha! There we go! Genetics schmenetics.

Hold up now, cowboy. While how we gain (or lose) weight is

indeed down to physics, the more complex question is why? Why do some people end up eating more than others? What we now know is that by studying the genetics of bodyweight, of which at one end of the spectrum sits obesity, we are by and large studying the genetics of how our brains influence our feeding behaviour. Many of us, for a myriad of different biological reasons, are more drawn towards food than others; in effect, some of us find it more difficult to say 'no' than others.

Our bodyweight is not a choice.

But surely you are choosing to put that slice of pizza or burger or cookie in your mouth? OK, sure, any given food decision is binary: do I eat this cookie or not? But realise that we don't gain or (sadly) lose weight overnight. Our bodyweight is the function of many thousands of binary food decisions over many years. So imagine if because of your genes, you are 5 per cent less likely to be able to say 'no'; for instance, if you manage to say 'no' nineteen times in a row, but the twentieth time comes along and the choice is some really great Chicago-style deep-dish pizza or not, and then you say, hang it, I'll have that slice of pizza. Over many thousands of food decisions, that is potentially thousands of extra calories, which is why some of us are, as in the tale of Goldilocks, too small, too large, or just right. That is the nuance of the system. If it is more difficult to say 'no', you will inevitably end up eating more than someone else who finds it easier to say 'no'. And if it is more difficult to say 'no', then is it really a choice?

As with many other human traits, some of the key observations that revealed the powerful role of genetics in bodyweight were made through the study of twins. The concept of 'twin studies' as a tool for the study of human traits is simple yet tremendously powerful. As we know, there are identical twins and non-identical twins. Identical twins are the result of one fertilised egg that splits into two before each going on to fully develop within the womb, so they are, in effect, genetic clones. Non-identical twins are the result of two different eggs being fertilised by two different sperm at the same time, which then go on to develop into babies, thus they share as much genetic material as you do with your own siblings, or for that matter your folks, so 50 per cent. You can take any given human trait and ask how similar it is when you share 100 per cent of genes versus 50 per cent of genes, and work out what geneticists refer to as 'heritability', which is the percentage of the variation of a given trait that can be explained by genetics as opposed to the environment. For example, if I had hair, it would be black, and I would argue that hair colour is very powerfully genetically determined, with very little environment impact (peroxide or dye does not count). Whereas, while the ability to have freckles is undoubtedly genetically influenced, how many and if they appear, even between identical twins, would depend on whether you like the sun, or wear T-shirts. So there we have an example of a genetic trait with an equally powerful environmental influence.

In 1986, Albert Stunkard and his colleagues from the University of Pennsylvania School of Medicine in Philadelphia studied 1974 identical and 2097 non-identical twin pairs in order to calculate the heritability of height, weight and BMI.[6] Stunkard found that concordance rates for bodyweight were twice as high for identical twins as for non-identical twins, and that heritability for height, weight, and BMI were 80 per cent, 78 per cent and 77 per cent respectively. That is to say, identical twins had similar bodyweights, which suggests there is a genetic component to what we weigh. This was, particularly for bodyweight, surprisingly high. The issue with this initial study was that the vast majority of the twin pairs studied had, unsurprisingly, been raised in the same household. How then to separate out the shared environment of being raised together? We live in a world where, sadly, awful things can sometimes happen; one of which is that siblings, a percentage of whom will of course be twins, are sometimes separated at birth and raised by different adoptive parents, often in completely different countries and cultures. Then twenty-five years later, when they finally meet again on *Oprah*, it is a shock to everyone, often including themselves, how similar they are in their mannerisms and in their look. Well, in 1990, Stunkard repeated the study, but this time on hundreds of twin pairs that had been raised apart, and found that the heritability for BMI of identical twins reared apart was around 70 per cent.[7] Further studies performed by others, which both expanded on the numbers of twins and the circumstances in which they were raised, established the heritability of BMI to range between 40 per cent and 70 per cent. This means that between 40 per cent and 70 per cent of our differences in weight can be explained by our genes, with the inverse also being true, that 30 per cent to 60 per cent of our weight can be explained by the environment.

WHEN SUSCEPTIBLE GENES MEET A HIGH-RISK ENVIRONMENT

A question I am often asked when quoting the 40 per cent to 70 per cent figure for heritability of BMI is, why the broad range? Is it 40 per cent or is it 70 per cent? Well, what is certain is that every single human behaviour and characteristic will have a genetic component. The really tricky part is figuring out how much of a role the environment plays in the development and manifestation of each trait. With all of the technical wizardry now at our disposal, our ability to obtain genetic information is no longer a bottleneck, and the expertise and computing power required to effectively handle and analyse these data are rapidly becoming accessible to most scientists. Our genes also don't change, and they are what they are from the day we are born till the day we die. The environment, however, is a far trickier customer to get a handle on; it is

volatile, changes throughout our lives, and is therefore very difficult to measure, certainly at scale. To be a geneticist is not only to
study genes in isolation (well, you could, but it wouldn't give you
the complete story), but it is also to understand how the genes
interact and respond to the world around us. While the sequence
of our genes remains static throughout our lives, their expression,
the level to which they are turned on or off, changes constantly in
response to the shifting environment of life. So why 40 per cent to
70 per cent heritability rather than 100 per cent? Because of the
different environments that we all live in.

A clear demonstration of the powerful environmental influence
on the heritability of BMI was provided by my colleague Dr Clare
Llewellyn and her team at University College London. Llewellyn
runs the Gemini study, a population-based birth cohort of 2402
families with twins born in England and Wales between March
and December 2007.[8] It was set up to assess both genetic and
environmental contributions to early life growth, with a focus
on behavioural pathways. However, a crucial element to the
Gemini cohort is that for 925 of the participating twin pairs, of
which one third are identical, there are measures of the household
'risk for obesity'. This so-called 'obesogenic' risk was determined
by a detailed phone interview, and included information on the
availability and accessibility of fruit, vegetables, energy-dense
snacks and sugar-sweetened drinks; details of parental feeding
practices; as well as opportunities for physical activity and access
to (media) screens within the household. Llewellyn and her team
then integrated this information into a composite 'risk score'.
What Llewellyn and her team found was the heritability of BMI
was 86 per cent among children living in overall HIGHER-risk
home environments. Remember that these twins are in a family
unit and have been raised in the same household, not apart, thus
the high heritability. However, the really eye-opening finding,
particularly for the geneticist in me, was that for those living in

overall LOWER-risk home environments, their BMI heritability was only 39 per cent![9] Gemini is a birth cohort, meaning that all twins (or as many as possible in reality) born during a particular period were recruited; this is in contrast, for example, to a disease cohort, where people are recruited with a given disease so it can be studied. Thus, Gemini is broadly reflective of the English and Welsh populations in 2007, and there should be, on average, no genetic difference between the twins living in the higher-risk environment and those living in the lower-risk environment. What the study tells us is that even if you have been dealt a genetic hand of cards that makes you more susceptible to being obese, a healthier environment more than halves the risk of you becoming overweight, while being exposed to a less healthy environment maximises your genetic burden. This experiment illustrates why there is the 40 per cent to 70 per cent range for the heritability of BMI.

Basically, if you find it more difficult to say 'no', then it is naturally better to be in situations where you are not forced to make the decision in the first place. These results suggest that modifying the home environment, probably the only part of the environment we have any control over, could be effective in preventing weight gain in those genetically at risk for obesity. This is particularly important for susceptible children, as many studies have shown that those that are overweight or obese when young are far more likely to stay overweight or obese as adults.

But that, however, is easier said than done.

TOO LITTLE OF WHAT THEY NEED AND TOO MUCH OF WHAT THEY DON'T NEED

The 2020 review on Health Equity in England by Sir Michael Marmot revealed some startling statistics.[10] In the aftermath of the 2008 global financial crisis there had been widespread austerity measures, with deep cuts in most areas of public spending. Government spending as a percentage of GDP declined by 7 per cent between 2010 and 2019, from 42 per cent to 35 per cent. The brunt of these cuts were born by local authorities, which suffered a 77 per cent drop in funding from central government. In addition, spending on social protection and education declined by 1.5 per cent of GDP. Now, cuts are clearly never welcomed, but sometimes they are necessary. However, how and where they have fallen has been shown to be both regressive and inequitable; they have been greatest in areas of deprivation where need is highest. Sir Michael also cast his view on ethnicity, recognising that it intersects with socioeconomic position to produce particularly poor outcomes for some minority ethnic groups. For example, the latest annual report by the Social Metrics Commission found that nearly half of Black African Caribbean households were in poverty, compared with just under one in five white families, while BAME (Black, Asian and Minority Ethnicity) families as a whole were between two and three times as likely to be in persistent poverty than white households.

All of this matters because levels of deprivation are closely linked to health. Life expectancy at birth for males living in the most deprived areas in England was 73.9 years between 2016 and 2018, compared with 83.4 years in the least deprived areas; the corresponding figures for females were 78.6 and 86.3 years. That is a ten-year difference entirely based on deprivation. While life expectancy is clearly a critical measure of health, how long a person can expect to live in good health and therefore have quality of life is even more important. On average, healthy life expectancy at birth differs by twelve years between the most- and least-deprived local authorities for men and women. Thus the Marmot review concluded that the cuts have harmed health and contributed to widening health inequalities in the short-term and are likely to continue to do so over the longer term.

One of the most important drivers of inequality emerging from deprivation is access to a healthy diet. And the ones in society that are impacted most of all by malnutrition are (and have always been) children. The 2019 UNICEF report on childhood malnutrition zeroes in on the existential question at hand:

'*Why are so many children eating too little of what they need, while an increasing number of children are eating too much of what they don't need?*'[11]

UNICEF's definition of malnutrition isn't simply a matter of not getting enough to eat. Today it can be considered as three different, but often overlapping, problems: undernutrition, hidden hunger and being overweight. Undernutrition, as the name suggests, is not getting enough to eat, and so is the traditional definition of malnutrition. Hidden hunger refers to deficiencies in vitamins and other essential nutrients, including not getting enough protein and fibre; it is referred to as 'hidden' because it is often not visible, particular in its early stages. As for being overweight, people think of that as a result of too much good nutrition (such as in my house in lockdown . . .), which for some it undoubtedly is. However, there are many underprivileged kids who are overweight and obese because of over-consumption of foods that are energy dense, high in fat, sugar and salt, yet low in protein and fibre, and therefore also suffer from hidden hunger. Thus, malnutrition in children must now be considered against a backdrop of rapid change, including the growth of urban populations and the globalisation of food systems, which is leading to increased availability of food that is high in calories but low in nutrients, largely the 'ultra-processed' foods we were discussing in the last chapter. The bottom line is, malnutrition today, in all its forms, is driven by the poor quality of children's diets, with two thirds of children in the world not being fed the minimum recommended diverse diet for healthy growth and development. Two in every three children! If there was ever any doubt, this is not a niche issue.

Folks, I'm not trying to be a downer just for the hell of it. If we don't acknowledge this unequivocal link between deprivation, malnutrition and diet-related disease, we will not be able to sort any of these problems out. The greatest tragedy of all is that malnutrition, as is true with most disease, is shouldered by children and young people from the poorest and most marginalised communities, creating a vicious cycle and perpetuating poverty across generations. This should be unacceptable to all of us in the twenty-first century.

PRIVILEGE IS HAVING CHOICES

But if people are hungry, shouldn't they be skinny? If they are having problems with weight, then surely they can't be hungry? I think it is all about bad choices, really . . . I mean, look, they are eating at those awful fast-food places! Why are they buying all that ultra-processed junk? Look at what they are feeding those kids, I mean, it is shocking. Don't they know what goes into those cheap sausage rolls and chicken nuggets? Why buy frozen pizzas when it is so easy to make your own? Don't they care about their children? If that's what they are eating then they deserve to be unhealthy! They just need to cook from scratch so they know what goes into their food! They need to shop at farmers' markets, and grow their own as much as possible, so they know what goes into their food. Organic is key for health, really. Vegetables and beans and lentils are cheap and nutritious, after all!

These are just a flavour of the comments that people have chosen to say out loud to me (as I've said previously, I have a sharing face). Trust me when I say I have overheard much worse and couched in far more derogatory terms.

Jane and I are both on academic salaries, live in a reasonably sized house, drive regular cars, eat out every so often, and fly economy class when we go on vacation (sometimes we splash out on 'premium economy' ... ooooh), and if either of us lost our jobs, it wouldn't be too long before we'd be in trouble paying our mortgage. We are typically 'middle-class' and, at the risk of making sweeping assumptions, this is probably some variation of the situations most of you reading this book find yourself in. We lead comfortable lives and are most definitely steeped in privilege. While the link between deprivation and undernutrition is understandable to most, it is counter-intuitive to many people – the overwhelming majority of whom are privileged – that deprivation can possibly be linked to being overweight and obesity.

Privilege comes in three different flavours: money, time and knowledge. Earning enough money is the first thing that comes to mind when we speak of privilege, and obviously is very much at the heart of the issue. How about having enough time? Well, Mrs Smith might make enough money to feed her family and pay the rent, but maybe she needs to hold down two minimum-wage jobs, one full-time, and one weekends and evenings, in order to do so; thus Mrs Smith has just enough money to survive, but no time to do anything else. And finally there is having access to knowledge. Does Mrs Smith, for example, have the money or time to access information about what foods are high in vitamin C, or iodine, or fibre? To know how much is too much sugar? To understand the difference between saturated and unsaturated fat? Does she know what a pulse is, or what tofu is made from, or where gluten is found? The lower down the socioeconomic ladder one goes, the more deprived one is, and the less of all three flavours of privilege one is likely to have.

I don't have to worry about where my next meal is coming from. On the one hand, if I choose to cook, I have enough disposable income to procure just the right ingredients, as well as time and knowledge to be able to produce a nutritious meal, from scratch, for the family. If I don't want to cook, I can choose to eat out or get a Deliveroo or Uber Eats delivery. I have the resources to make these choices.

Mrs Smith, more often than not, does not have that luxury.

In 2019, just prior to the publication of his 2020 review on Health Equity in England, Sir Michael Marmot gave an interview to the 'Health Service Journal'. In it he said:

'If everyone followed Public Health England's eating advice, people in the bottom decile (10 per cent) of household income would spend 74 per cent of their income on food. So, there's not much point telling them to follow the healthy eating advice they can't afford.'[12]

Sir Michael is clear people should take personal responsibility for their health. However:

'You can't expect people to take responsibility for feeding their children healthy food if they're in the bottom 10 per cent of household income and can't afford to buy healthy food. Or . . . if they're one of the million people who go off to food banks.'

And that is why the type of food environment we live in is crucial. Today, many healthy 'unprocessed' foods are more expensive than their ultra-processed counterparts. For example, in the experiment discussed in Chapter 7, comparing the effects of an unprocessed versus the equivalent ultra-processed diet, the authors of the study estimated that the weekly cost for ingredients to prepare 2000kcal a day of ultra-processed meals was, in US dollars, $106 versus $151 for the unprocessed meals;[13] nearly a third less. Ultra-processed meals, because of the industrial scale at which they are manufactured, ease of transport and long shelf-life, are simply cheaper to the consumer in terms of cost per calorie.

Then there is the issue with the proliferation of takeaway vendors and fast-food restaurants. Please don't get me wrong; I love chicken nuggets or fried chicken or burgers and fries or pizza as much as anyone else. However, while takeaway numbers have increased over the years in many places, it is where they have demonstrated the fastest rate of growth that is particularly eye-opening. Scientists from the University of Cambridge did a study examining the number and location of takeaway food outlets in the county of Norfolk, which is in the East of England, from 1990 to 2008.[14] Over the eighteen-year period, the number of takeaway food outlets rose by 45 per cent, from 2.6 outlets to 3.8 outlets per 10,000 residents in the county as a whole. When they broke the numbers down by postal code, however, they found that the areas of least deprivation saw an increase from 1.6 outlets to 2.1 outlets per 10,000 residents (a 30 per cent increase), whereas the areas of highest deprivation saw an increase from 4.6 outlets to 6.5 outlets per 10,000 residents (a 43 per cent increase). Further studies have shown similar trends throughout the rest of the UK. Nationwide, there are two to three times as many takeaways in the most-deprived areas, where their growth has been concentrated, compared to the least-deprived areas.[15] Why has this happened? Well, takeaway food can represent a very low-cost option to the consumer, with £1 in some places able to purchase as many as 900 calories! With national data showing that children living in areas surrounded by fast-food outlets are more likely to be overweight or obese, is the presence of takeaways the result of demand, causing the problem, or both? These studies are not set up to answer questions of causality, but with takeaway consumption associated with a greater increase in total calorie consumption for children in lower socio-economic groups than children in higher socio-economic groups, it is fair to say their location is likely to be contributing to inequalities in diet and bodyweight.

CHECK YOUR PRIVILEGE

For many, the 'healthy' option is simply not affordable or convenient. If you have less money, and you really haven't the time or any idea how to quickly assemble a meal, from scratch, to feed the kids, then you are going to have to make the choices that you have to make. People are not deprived because they make poor choices. Deprivation leads to poor 'choices' or, more often than not, no choices.

This is something that those in the world of diet and nutrition might well remember when trying to push (push being the operative word here) certain dietary approaches. Evangelical vegans or plant-based gurus are a case in point. There is a huge distinction between being vegetarian and being vegan. For much of human history, we were probably largely vegetarian, eating very little meat, if only because meat was expensive. Keeping in mind that we never had enough food to eat (the last thirty to forty years being the exception), could you really afford to eat the cow if it could produce milk, or the chicken if it was laying eggs? Because of milk and eggs, being vegetarian is naturally nutritionally complete and can actually be a very economical way to eat. Anyone can be vegetarian if they choose. Being vegan, however, is complicated, because you will have to take supplements if you want to be healthy. I've expressed this opinion many times on various social media outlets (sucker for punishment, I know), and I've always received significant blowback. Arguments include: it is easy, people just have to watch their pulses and supplements (listen to yourself); don't the animals get a say? (I am all for eating ethically, and those of us who can choose to should); there is no safe dose of animal protein (there is – it is true that the privileged in society are eating too much meat, and we certainly need to eat less, but there is a safe dose of animal protein). Being vegan is certainly a *choice* that some of us are in the position to make, and it is certainly a healthy choice if done correctly. This holds true for many of the other diets I've discussed in this book. But please remember to check your privilege. We shouldn't foist our privileged choice on others who don't have a choice.

WE CAN'T CHANGE OUR GENES BUT WE CAN (TRY TO) FIX SOCIETY

Obesity and other diet-related illnesses are indeed serious public-health crises that have been, to date, intractable at a population level to any effective long-term interventions. A big part of the reason is because obesity is still believed, by most of society, including policy makers and government, to be a 'lifestyle' disease. Obesity is considered to be the result of bad decisions, the result of poor choices.

There is a big difference between pointing out a problem that needs solving, and blaming the people suffering from the problem. For instance, I have described, from a genetic and biological perspective, why bodyweight is not a choice. In this chapter, however, I have, hopefully, also demonstrated that our socioeconomic status plays nearly as big a role! A difference between a 40 per cent heritability of BMI amongst the most privileged and an 80 per cent heritability amongst the least privileged.

Take THAT to the bank.

We can't change our genes, either technically or ethically, at least for now. Poverty and deprivation, however, is something that we should absolutely refuse to accept. With the right political and societal will, it is a solvable problem.

Don't let anybody tell you otherwise.

CHAPTER 9

We don't eat calories, we eat food

'If you focus on health, your weight will take care of itself.'

Me

Bodyweight, for myriad different biological and societal reasons, is not a choice. But that doesn't mean that obesity is not an existential public-health issue. There is simply a big distinction between pointing out a problem and blaming the people suffering from the problem. The fact is, the vast majority of non-communicable diseases that are prevalent today are diet-related, and there are many people who do need to lose weight to reduce their risk of disease, and in some cases, even put certain diseases, type 2 diabetes in particular, into remission. Yet, at the same time, there are those who subscribe to 'body positivity', arguing that weight is simply a number that is used to batter people over the head who are overweight or living with obesity, and that there is health at every size.

SHOULD WE FEAR FAT OR SHOULD WE BE BODY POSITIVE?

The body-positivity movement was founded on the belief that all of us should have a positive body image and advocates the acceptance of all bodies regardless of physical ability, size, gender, race or appearance. I completely understand the emergence of body positivity as a response in protest to the overt 'fat-shaming' that is not only cruel but counter-productive and yet inexplicably ubiquitous in society. I certainly also believe that we should not judge people on how they look and how much they weigh. But let us just say that I am overweight and at a demonstrably higher risk of disease; is this something I'm compelled to accept? If I then choose to try and lose weight, does that mean I hate who I am now and no longer have a positive body image? What happens if I try to lose weight and, God forbid, actually succeed? Does that mean I don't accept others who haven't tried, or the many who have tried and failed?

I fear that some within the body-positivity movement have gone too far and are ignoring the science. What is unequivocal, and please don't shoot the messenger, is that carrying too much fat is bad for your health. This leads to two questions: why is fat bad for you, and how much is too much fat?

First, why is fat considered to be bad? Because, in large part, people misunderstand what happens when they gain or lose weight; they think that they are gaining fat cells or losing fat cells, hence that they are bad and need to be got rid of. This is not true. You have to consider your fat cells, also known as adipocytes, like balloons; they get bigger when you gain weight, and they get smaller when you lose weight. The actual number of your adipocytes doesn't change by much at all. Now, the safest place to store fat is in the form of triglycerides within the adipocytes; all of our adipocytes together form our professional fat-storage organ, and are our key long-term energy reservoir. Depending on individual size, humans can have between 90,000 and 180,000 calories of fat stored on board at any time. Thus fat, per se, is not bad for you, and the much-maligned adipocytes are certainly not evil and they need to be fully appreciated for the crucial role they play. However, like all balloons, adipocytes will expand until they can't expand any more, but unlike balloons, they don't pop (thank goodness).

This is when the trouble begins, because once our adipocyte stores are full, then the fat has to go somewhere else, and ends up in our muscles or our liver, for example. While muscles and the liver are designed to store some fat, too much fat begins to adversely affect their function, in a phenomenon known as 'lipotoxicity', literally meaning fat poisoning. Thus, it is only when we are carrying more than we can safely store that fat becomes toxic, and that is when we tilt into diseases such as type 2 diabetes, heart disease and certain cancers.[1]

OK, then how much is too much fat? When does it become dangerous? So here is the interesting thing: depending on our individual biology, our fat cells are able to expand to different sizes before becoming full. So East Asian (such as Chinese folk like me) and South Asian (such as Indians, Pakistanis and Bangladeshis) people don't have to put on that much weight before increasing their risk of getting type 2 diabetes, for example. Whereas other ethnicities, including white people and, famously, Polynesians for example, can gain a lot more weight before becoming ill, in large part, due to the expandability of their adipocytes.[2]

Another important characteristic that influences our susceptibility to disease is our body shape, which is, in effect, where we put our fat. Are you big in the middle, but have relatively skinny arms and legs, so-called 'apple' shaped? Do you perhaps have a big bum and legs, with a smaller top, so-called 'pear' shaped? Or are you large all over and sorta look like a sausage? An apple-shaped person is typically, although not exclusively, male, and has accumulated a lot of fat around their organs. This type of fat is also known as visceral fat and tends to result in a large but tight stereotypical 'beer-belly' (hello, Jack). A pear-shaped individual is typically, although not exclusively, female, and carries fat primarily around the bum, arms and legs, so called subcutaneous fat. Why should you care about where your fat goes? Because apple-shaped people, who therefore carry more visceral fat, are at a higher risk of metabolic disease. And because men tend to carry more visceral fat then women, they in turn have a higher risk of developing heart disease and other metabolic problems.

Our body shape and the degree to which our fat cells can expand are both powerful genetically influenced traits and inform our differing safe fat-carrying capacities. So in any given population there is most definitely health present at many possible sizes; with some larger folk being the picture of metabolic health, and other lean and fit-looking people with type 2 diabetes. But here is the critical take-home message: for any given individual, there cannot be health at every size, because if you surpass your own safe fat-carrying capacity, you WILL become ill. I am not saying this to be body negative, and I am certainly not judging or blaming anyone who chooses not to lose weight, or who has tried and been unsuccessful. I am simply stating a crystal-clear biological fact.

Given the food environment we are living in today, and with the prevalence of obesity as high as it is, there are many people who are at the edge of their safe fat-carrying capacity. The ability to determine a person's fat-carrying capacity is the subject of cutting-edge genetic and biological research, and would be a game-changer, transforming the way we consider the definition of 'obesity' and who actually needs to lose weight. Until then, we can only identify the many who have blown right past their fat-carrying limit when they find themselves in a state of disease.

WHAT IS THE BEST WAY TO LOSE WEIGHT?

So returning to Jack and Diane, our favourite couple from the introduction, you will recall that they had just received the loud and clear message from their doctor that regardless of the difficulty, they really need to lose weight in order to improve their health. What are they to do? Sadly, if you made it this close to the end of the book in hope of me sharing some magical solution, a silver bullet, then I fear you will be disappointed. There is no magic and there are no shortcuts. The only way that Jack and Diane, and anyone else for that matter, will lose weight is by creating a 'calorie deficit'; they will need to reduce the number of calories they are eating.

Now, hang on, I hear the peanut-eating sceptics say, the title of this book is literally *Why Calories Don't Count*, and now you're asking us to count calories? We want our money back!

I'm not asking anyone to count calories at all, because the number of calories, simply taken in isolation, and out of context from whence they came, is not a particularly useful piece of information. Don't get me wrong, calorie information does of course have its place. For one thing, calories are useful in quantifying portion sizes, so a 200-calorie portion of French fries will have twice the energy as a 100-calorie portion of fries. Also, calorie information at point of purchase, such as added to menus or put next to food in restaurants, coffee shops and cafeterias, does seem to give people pause for thought, and has been shown to reduce calories purchased by about 8 per cent per meal.[3] So eating fewer calories of fries, or not purchasing – and hence consuming – the muffin after seeing that it contained 400 calories would be examples of creating a 'calorie deficit'.

But surely the exercise side of the 'in and out' energy balance equation would also be equally effective in creating a 'calorie deficit'? Yes, exercise and other types of physical activity do have their role to play. However, there is plenty of evidence that increasing physical activity in and of itself, without addressing the food-intake side of the equation, is not an effective way of shedding the pounds.[4] The reason is that the numbers are simply stacked against physical activity. Let's take a typical chocolate bar, for instance, all of which are formulated to be around 240 calories. If I am feeling motivated, and I often am, I can snaffle down a Snickers bar (other ultra-processed confectionery items are available) in less than two minutes. Yet it will always take around twenty to thirty minutes plodding along on a treadmill to burn off 240 calories. Basically, we are evolved to consume calories faster than we can burn them; it is one of the key characteristics that has ensured our evolutionary success, otherwise we'd spend too long chowing down on food and risk becoming tiger food. Sure, it is of course in principle possible to lose weight by not reducing food intake and simply exercising more. Take elite endurance athletes like UK long-distance runner Sir Mo Farah, for example, who has to eat nearly 4000 calories a day when in training; or Tour de France cyclists who burn through an average of 5000 calories per stage of the twenty-one-stage race yet still lose weight during the Tour because they literally don't have enough time in the day to eat and replenish all of the calories they have expended. For mere mortals like the most of us, however, our energy efficiency means that we simply don't run or cycle or do anything else tiring for long enough to achieve that! There is, on the other hand, good evidence of exercise being useful in helping to maintain weight after you've lost it. But, and it is a very important but, exercise is good for you, *independent of any weight loss*.[5] Being physically active lowers all-cause mortality and can prevent the onset of obesity, type 2 diabetes, hypertension, and cardiovascular disease. So everybody who is able should be encouraged to exercise or be physically active, regardless of the weight loss achieved or not achieved.

Thus, and at the risk of sounding like a broken record, the most effective way to lose weight is still to eat less. But wait, I hear you say, are you saying that I have to go on a diet? I thought they (whoever 'they' are) say that 95 per cent of diets don't work? Well, that is not technically true. Any diet that gets you to eat less, hence creating a 'calorie deficit', is a diet that works. The problem is, once you come off the diet, the weight, for the vast majority of people, comes piling back on. So a more accurate statement is that 95 per cent of diets we can't stick to. Losing weight (which is the easier part of the process) and keeping it off (this is undoubtedly the more difficult part) requires a long-term change to one's eating behaviour and patterns. That implies a number of things. First, whatever approach that you choose can't be extreme, because by definition 'extreme' would not be sustainable; second, it has got to suit your biology, which then gives it the best chance of working; and third, it has got to suit your life situation – so what can you afford? Do you have kids? Do you work shifts? How do you get to work? Because if it doesn't suit your lifestyle and situation, you will never be able to stick with it.

Given everything we have discussed in this book, let me show you, and all of the Jacks and Dianes out there, a few tips on how to leverage the 'caloric availability' concept in your day-to-day life, and empower yourselves to make healthier food choices. Just to be clear, this is not a 'plan'; there are no lists of instructions, no rules to stick to, and nothing to abstain from. Rather, consider this a strategy to help you navigate today's food environment.

COUNTING CALORIES

So why not count calories, like advocated by Lulu Hunt Peters, whom we were introduced to in Chapter 2? Because, calorie counting as a diet-plan, like needing to stick rigidly to a fixed number of calories per day, for instance, simply makes no sense without taking into account what foods they are coming from and their caloric availability. How do we then make sense of calorie information in the real world?

Go to your kitchen and grab any package of food that has front- and back-of-pack nutritional info and you will likely find that the calorie information on display is still derived from Atwater's original 9 calories per gram of fat, 4 calories per gram of carb and

4 calories per gram of protein general factors. Just take the fat, carb and protein info on the packaging and do the simple maths and you'll see that it will add up to the displayed calorie-count. Sometimes, it doesn't add up exactly, but sorta gets close; and the reason for this is that, confusingly, some manufacturers mix in (randomly, as far as I can tell) use of the 'Atwater specific factors' as well. The 'Atwater specific factors' are a refinement to the general factors introduced in 1955 by Merrill and Watt,[6] taking into account the influence of the proportions of protein, fat and carbohydrates in a given food, as well as the presence of fibre, on its heat of combustion (to refresh your memory, this is the heat given off when the food is burnt in a bomb calorimeter). The problem is the system relies entirely on a series of tables containing very specific numbers, for example, the Atwater specific factors for hen's eggs are 9.02 calories/gram of fat, 3.68 calories/gram of carbs and 4.36 calories/gram of protein (see Appendix 1 for a selection of foods with their corresponding specific factors). If you do the maths then the total calorie-counts do end up slightly different, and are a more accurate reflection of the actual heat of combustion of that food. However, tables are inherently unwieldy to use and, at any rate, they were not comprehensive (how could they be), even back in 1955! Hence this is why Atwater's century-old general factors in their simplicity still predominate.

However, having survived the crash course on intermediary metabolism in Chapters 3 and 4 (you all get a gold star), we now know that the Atwater factors, both general and specific, are inaccurate, because they don't take into account diet-induced thermogenesis (DIT), which is the energy, given off as heat, that is required for the metabolism of food. Fat has a DIT value between 0 and 3 per cent, meaning that for every 100 metabolisable calories of fat, it will cost between 0 and 3 calories to process. The DIT value for carbohydrates is between 5 and 10 per cent, meaning that for every 100 metabolisable calories of carbs, it will cost between 5 and 10 calories to process. While protein has the highest DIT value at 15 and 30 per cent, meaning that for every 100 metabolisable calories of protein, it will cost between 15 and 30 calories to process.

Thus, what I am proposing here is a simple 'back of the envelope' method to improve the 9–4–4 system. It will still not be fully accurate as the proportions of the different macronutrients and the amount of fibre present, which is a signature unique to each food type, does influence caloric availability, hence the existence of the tables of 'specific factors', a selection of which can be found in Appendix 1, but it is a better reflection of the available 'net metabolisable energy' or NME. My suggestions are as follows:

9 calories per gram of **fat**

3.8 calories per gram of **sugar**

3.6 calories per gram of **complex carbs**.

3.2 calories per gram of **protein**.

Fat costs next to nothing in terms of heat to process, so the Atwater factor of **9 calories per gram of fat** remains accurate. I suggest lowering the Atwater 4 calories per gram of carbs by 5 per cent for sugars (**3.8 calories per gram of sugar**) and 10 per cent for complex carbs (**3.6 calories per gram of complex carbs**). Finally, for protein, I suggest lowering the Atwater of 4 calories per gram by 20 per cent (conservatively taking a lower mid-point value), thus taking the figure down to **3.2 calories per gram of protein**.

Just to be clear, I didn't invent this concept of 'net metabolisable energy'. It was actually proposed by Geoffrey Livesey in the *British Journal of Nutrition* in 2001.[7] However, it was ignored for one reason or another, or wasn't noticed . . . but either way, it clearly didn't gain any traction. So this is me picking up the baton and trying to push 'net metabolisable energy' into the conversation.

OK, so what would this mean in the real world?

Let's say you were at your favourite restaurant for dinner, and on the menu is a Caesar salad to start, steak frites (a lovely cut of fillet steak served with fries) with creamed horseradish sauce on the side for your main, and a gorgeous slice of the chocolate fudge cake for dessert. Let's run the numbers and see how they stack up (the detailed calorie calculations can be found in Appendix 2).

Starting with the salad, let's assume we have a 100-gram portion (I'm not a chef, so I'm sure someone will tell me if this is too much or too little!). A typical Caesar salad would have 16g fat (I know, right? It is always the dressing that gets you), 8g carbs and 5g protein, which using the Atwater factors results in 196 calories. Using my correction, it would be 189 calories, a difference of 7 calories or 3.5 per cent.

Then on to the main meal. Fillet steak is typically served as a 200-gram portion, which on average, raw, would be 46g of protein, 11g of fat and trace amounts of carbs (if it is cooked in butter mmmm . . . then the fat-count jumps by another 20g; but let's say in this scenario that this was done on a charcoal grill, arguably more tasty with a lot less saturated fat). The calorie-count for this piece of loveliness using the Atwater factors would be 283.5 calories. Using my correction, it would be 246.2 calories, which is a difference of 37.3 calories or 14.2 per cent.

But what is a steak without fries? It would be like Lennon without McCartney, a cowboy without sad songs, or a convertible without an ocean highway (I'll stop now, but if you can't tell, I love fries). Two hundred grams of French fries (that is certainly how much I would serve myself . . . stop judging) would be 9.5g fat, 50g carbs and 4.8g protein, which would be 304 Atwater calories; with the correction, 281 calories. That is a 23 calorie or 7.5 per cent difference. Let's assume 25g of horseradish sauce – to be honest, I would have tons more; I like a bit of steak with my horseradish, but there is already enough judging going on. That would be 12.7g fat, 2.5g carbs and 0.3g protein, which is 126 Atwater calories and 124.7 corrected calories; so only a sliver of a difference at 1.3 calories or 1 per cent.

And then to end the evening, what would life be without

chocolate cake? Let us say a 100g slice (once again, I've never weighed a chocolate cake, so who knows really . . . this is probably a teensy piece), which would have 16.7g of fat, 51.3g of carbs and 3.9g of protein. The Atwater count: 371 calories, and corrected, 354 calories; a difference of 17 calories or 4.6 per cent.

That is a pretty decent-sized meal at 1280 total Atwater calories, which corrects to 1195 calories, a difference of 85 calories, or 6.6 per cent. Now I know that this doesn't seem a great deal to concern ourselves over, but a 6.6 per cent caloric-availability discrepancy over a week works out to more than 1100 calories, so the numbers add up pretty quickly.

Also I am compelled to say that the point of this exercise is not to use these numbers to say, 'Yay! I can now eat 1100 more calories in a week and not gain any weight!' The food clearly hasn't changed, and when you eat more you will still gain weight. Rather, it allows you to better understand the amount of usable calories you can get out of a given food. You will see that the discrepancy between the Atwater and my corrected numbers fluctuates depending on the composition of the food, with the smallest difference seen with the sauce, which is composed largely of fat with some carbs, but little to no protein, and the largest difference found with the steak, which is the part of the meal with the largest proportion of protein. The carb-heavy components sit somewhere in the middle, and their caloric availability will differ depending on the proportions of complex-to-refined carbohydrates and the presence of fibre.

Thus, foods that have more protein, complex carbs and fibre, and are therefore less calorically available, will display a greater discrepancy as compared to foods high in sugar and fat. Perhaps you are now rolling your eyes and saying 'duh, of course, that is so obvious'. That may very well be the case, but what this correction for net metabolisable energy allows you to do is to measure it, to put a number on it, and hopefully be a useful tool to those hoping to improve their diet, and to others trying to achieve a calorie deficit.

WHAT IS THE BEST DIET?

Calorie counting aside, there are many people who, for one reason or another, are wedded to a particular diet approach. Now I am certainly not here to tell people how or how not to eat; if your approach works for you and your health, then you do you! Broadly speaking, there are three classes of diets that actually work, at least in the short-term, and at least for some people: those that directly get you to cut calories, and include (of course) calorie counting, as well as all varieties of intermittent fasting and time-restricted feeding; the 'low-carb, high-fat' #LCHF diets that we now know are almost all universally high in protein; and the largely, if not entirely, plant-based approaches. Now at this point I'm expecting some push-back from people saying that their diet works by some other obscure mechanism. What I'm saying is if you strip away the noise and take things back to their fundamental principles, you will find that your pet diet will almost certainly fit into one of these three categories. As you have found out in Chapters 5 and 6, the vast majority of diets in the latter two categories work to achieve a calorie deficit based on the principles of caloric availability. There are, however, some useful takeaways that can make your favourite approach better and possibly more sustainable.

For all you Keto fans out there, just remember that while it is effective in the short-term for weight-loss, there haven't been any long-term safety studies done, so once you have achieved whatever weight target you were aiming for, you may wish to consider introducing a moderate amount of healthy sources of carbohydrates, such as higher-fibre starchy foods, vegetables, fruit and legumes. One of the problems with Keto is that many find it hard to stick to because of the combination of high fat and ultra-low carb, so including some low-glycaemic-index carbohydrates could very well make sustaining a largely Keto approach possible both for palatability and health reasons, thus giving you the best chance of maintaining that weight loss. The other problem with Keto is that people end up eating too much red meat and saturated fat. Try to consume more white meat, or better still, fish, and shift to as much unsaturated fat as possible and make sure you get enough fibre. This advice holds true for all of the diets in the #LCHF emporium. Except for Carnivore; I'm not sure how people are sticking to a supposed 'Carnivore' Diet (which humans are most certainly not) and not keeling over and dying. Don't do Carnivore. There. After saying that I won't tell people how to eat, I will tell you to not do Carnivore.

Then on the other end of the dietary spectrum, there are the vegan and plant-based approaches (not to mention the whole shooting-match of randomly restrictive diets with ridiculously abstruse backstories, that are simply plant-based diets by another name) that are also effective for weight loss. There are certainly no problems with lack of fibre if you go down this route, but you do need to make sure you watch your protein needs. Tofu is a fabulous option if you like it (I love tofu), but otherwise eat as colourful an array of pulses as possible. Also, B12, iron, iodine, calcium and omega-3 supplementation is highly advised. For many, particularly if you are less privileged or cash-strapped, vegetarianism is a good option, because supplementation is not required.

My personal preference is one of moderation. What is clear is that we, the privileged in the world, need to eat less meat, particularly red meat, for both our health and the health of the planet. But meat, in moderation, can certainly play an important role in a healthy diet. My plant-based experiment that I detailed in Chapter 6 had a surprisingly large influence on my dietary mindset, and for over three years now I have been a 'flexitarian', whereby I am vegan during weekday lunches and at least twice a week in the evenings. I have probably cut my meat intake by 40 to 50 per cent and that can only be a good thing. Taking this approach has allowed me to keep off the weight, which I lost while I was fully plant-based, and yet is sustainable in the long-term, certainly for me.

NAVIGATING AN 'ULTRA-PROCESSED' WORLD

Finally, what should the strategy be in handling ultra-processed foods? The main issue is in many high-income countries, including the UK, most of Europe, most Australasian countries and the USA, ultra-processed foods now provide more than 50 per cent of the calories we consume. I certainly think we should be limiting the consumption of certain classes of ultra-processed foods. However, given their ubiquity, it is actually quite hard, if not impossible, to completely avoid them. It is also particularly unhelpful, I find, to tell someone to replace a chocolate bar, say, with a banana, or to replace crisps with celery and hummus dip. For one thing, these are not equivalent replacements! Sometimes you want a banana, but other times life demands a chocolate bar! If you have bought or even homemade hummus in your fridge to be served with crudités (hello, all you middle-class people, I am looking at you), then rock on; but sometimes what you really crave is a big bag of crisps. In addition, one has to remember that while some of us might be privileged enough to choose not to eat ultra-processed food, there are many for whom, because of their life situation, ultra-processed food is the cheapest option to feed themselves and their families. There is certainly an urgent debate to be had about the role of 'ultra-processed' in our food system and how it might be driving health inequalities; but please remember to check your privilege before judging, in fact, best not to judge at all.

I also think that rather than demonise the companies that manufacture and supply the many ultra-processed foods, we would be better in engaging with them to improve the nutritional profile of their products. Just from a purely commercial perspective, and maybe I am naïve in thinking this, surely we can impress upon food companies that if they make healthier food, we would stay alive for longer to spend more money with them? Anyway, in the meantime, my view is we have to be pragmatic and have strategies to navigate a largely ultra-processed world. Put simply, if you are in a chocolate-bar or frozen-pizza type of mood, can you choose a better chocolate bar or pizza?

This, I think, is an easy win. It is important to realise that not all ultra-processed products are created equal, and we can try to make better decisions by simply looking at the ingredients list, and picking foods that are higher in protein and fibre, and lower in sugar, salt and fat.

Take two different ultra-processed frozen lasagnes, for example, the nutritional values for a 100g portion of which I have extracted for you in the table opposite. On the left is a lasagne made with regular pasta, and to the right, a lasagne containing whole-wheat pasta (yes, they exist!). The calorie-counts, which come from the manufacturers, would have been calculated using the Atwater specific factors, rather than the general factors. Importantly, you will notice that while the whole-wheat lasagne contains a similar amount of sugar and more fat (3g vs 1.79g), it has, crucially, 2.5g more protein and 6.4g more fibre per 100g portion. The same class of frozen ultra-processed lasagne, costing the same amount, yet with such a difference in nutritional content! If you are in a chocolate-bar type of mood, then ones that contain nuts (as long as you are not allergic) will often have more protein; and others that have dried fruit in will contain a higher percentage of fibre. The numbers are here for all of us to see (sometimes requiring the use of reading glasses); just check it out next time you are at a physical supermarket or shopping online.

Lasagne			Whole-wheat Lasagne		
Name	Amount	Unit	Name	Amount	Unit
Energy	357	kcal	Energy	320	kcal
Protein	12.5	g	Protein	14	g
Total lipid (fat)	1.79	g	Total lipid (fat)	3	g
Carbohydrate, by difference	75	g	Carbohydrate, by difference	70	g
Fibre, total dietary	3.6	g	Fibre, total dietary	10	g
Sugars, total	3.57	g	Fibre, soluble	2	g
			Fibre, insoluble	10	g
			Sugars, total	4	g

WE DON'T EAT CALORIES, WE EAT FOOD

So there we have it, my meditation on 'the calorie', that most misunderstood and misused of units of energy. I have taken you through its history, from its inception as a niche measure used primarily by scientists, all the way to its weaponisation by the diet industry. I have described how our body digests and metabolises food to extract the calories locked up within and detailed what we use the calories for. Somewhere along the way, in thinking about the science of weight loss, however, we forgot that we don't eat calories, we eat food. Why don't calories count? Because the number of calories in a food does not reflect the type of food or the quality of food. A number doesn't take into account the physiological responses of our body to certain types of foods, such as protein being more satiating, and fibre keeping our bowels, our symbiotic gut microbiome and hence our whole being in a healthy and happy state. Count calories all you want, but used as a cold hard number, all a calorie-count does is reflect the amount of a given type of food.

But when we treat calories with a bit more nuance, when we understand that where they come from makes a huge difference to their availability and how our body responds and deals with them, then calories very much have their place. I have explained that the principles of caloric availability underlie how most popular diets work, as well as why consumption of ultra-processed foods is linked to increased bodyweight. The two biggest factors that influence the availability of calories in food are protein and fibre content, and it just so happens that these two factors also play important roles in the quality of our diet and our overall health. Thus, I hope that this newfound understanding of caloric availability can empower you to make better decisions about your diet, to be able to leverage this information to eat better and possibly even create a calorie deficit so you can shed some pounds . . . if you need to, that is.

But do remember that while today weight is used almost universally as a proxy for health – hence all the noise around calories, and what drove me to write this book – when taken in isolation and out of context of all other physiological measures it is of limited utility. One's weight, sadly, is also almost universally used as a proxy for beauty. So here is my final thought: rather than wasting our lives obsessing about our weight and how we look, we should, instead, focus on our health.

If you focus on health, your weight will take care of itself.

And that, as they say, is that. It was a pleasure having all of you along for the ride.

EPILOGUE

WHAT TO COUNT INSTEAD OF CALORIES?

Before I sat down to write this epilogue, I went onto YouTube to watch the video for John Mellencamp's 'Jack and Diane' again; for inspiration, you understand.

First of all, the song is still as awesome as I remembered, and second, they were most definitely young, skinny and pretty in the video. I guess the question is, if I were Jack and Diane's (the late-forties version from the introduction) doctor, and they had come to me for help, what would I say? Well, first, I wouldn't have brought up their future grandkids (it is indeed a low blow, and once you've lost your audience, they will no longer listen to you), and second, I most certainly would not have asked them to count calories. While it is true that we need to eat fewer calories if we want to lose weight, as I've argued in this book, simply blindly counting calories makes little sense.

OK, Mr Negative, I hear many of you saying, how about some practical solutions instead? How about some useful advice for once?

Oof, low blow.

Well, I guess if Jack and Diane were to ask my advice on how to be healthier, this is what I'd tell them: hang the calories and pay more attention to the nutritional content of your food. I am always hesitant to offer overly prescriptive advice, as we are all so different and have varying nutritional needs, but if you focus your counting attention elsewhere, rather than on calories, you will be making healthier food choices by default. Think about eating enough protein, more fibre, less sugar and less meat.

PROTEIN ~ 16 PER CENT OF YOUR DAILY ENERGY INTAKE

Remember that there is a 'sweet spot' for the amount of protein. And that spot is around 16 per cent of your daily energy intake. Please also remember that protein doesn't only mean meat, but can come from a wide range of plant-based sources. Also, try to eat more white meat and fish, and less red and processed meats. A portion of cooked meat would be 60 to 90 grams, famously about the size of a deck of cards. Whereas a portion of cooked white or oily fish, which is less nutritionally dense than (land-based) meat, is 140 grams, or a piece around the size of the palm of your hand. If you are vegetarian, you would need to eat 180 to 200 grams of tofu, or perhaps 200 grams each of chickpeas and green peas.

FIBRE > 30 GRAMS PER DAY

Consider 30 grams a day a minimum amount. This is nowhere close to the 50 grams a day suggested by Denis Burkitt, but is far more than the average of 16 to 18 grams a day that we in high-income countries are currently achieving. What would this look like? Well, a couple of slices of wholemeal bread contains 5 grams of fibre, 100 grams of broccoli has 2.3 grams of fibre, 100 grams of peas has 4.5 grams of fibre, and 100 grams of almonds has 7.4

grams of fibre. So if you ate all of that, that would be nearly 20 grams of fibre, which is more than we are eating now, and two thirds our way to 30 grams a day! But the more the better really.

FREE SUGARS < 5 PER CENT OF YOUR DAILY ENERGY INTAKE

'Free sugars' are sugars that are not inside the cells of the food we eat. This obviously includes the powdered or granulated form of sugar. However, while it doesn't refer to sugar in whole fruit, it does include the sugar in fruit juice, from which the fibre has been removed. Free sugars also refer to that found in honey, syrups and nectars.

MEAT-FREE DAYS

We do need to eat less meat and more plants, both for our health and for the environment. I hesitate to be overly prescriptive about this, but perhaps aim for one to two meat-free days a week, or one meat-free meal per day, or even both, if it floats your boat!

Remember, we eat food, not calories, and if you take care of your health, your weight will take care of itself.
Peace and out.

APPENDIX 1

Selected Atwater Specific Factors

	Protein kcal/g (kJ/g)	Fat kcal/g (kJ/g)	Carbohydrate kcal/g (kJ/g)
Eggs, meat products, milk products:			
Eggs	4.36 (18.2)	9.02 (37.7)	3.68 (15.4)
Meat/fish	4.27 (17.9)	9.02 (37.7)	*
Milk/milk products	4.27 (17.9)	8.79 (36.8)	3.87 (16.2)
Fats – separated:			
Butter	4.27 (17.9)	8.79 (36.8)	3.87 (16.2)
Margarine, vegetable	4.27 (17.9)	8.84 (37.0)	3.87 (16.2)
Other vegetable fats and oils	–	8.84 (37.0)	–
Fruits:			
All, except lemons, limes	3.36 (14.1)	8.37 (35.0)	3.60 (15.1)
Fruit juice, except lemon, lime	3.36 (14.1)	8.37 (35.0)	3.92 (15.1)
Lemon, limes	3.36 (14.1)	8.37 (35.0)	2.48 (10.4)
Lemon juice, lime juice	3.36 (14.1)	8.37 (35.0)	2.70 (11.3)
Grain products:			
Barley, pearled	3.55 (14.9)	8.37 (35.0)	3.95 (16.5)
Cornmeal, whole ground	2.73 (11.4)	8.37 (35.0)	4.03 (16.9)
Macaroni, spaghetti	3.91 (16.4)	8.37 (35.0)	4.12 (17.2)
Oatmeal (rolled oats)	3.46 (14.5)	8.37 (35.0)	4.12 (17.2)
Rice, brown	3.41 (14.3)	8.37 (35.0)	4.12 (17.2)
Rice, white or polished	3.82 (16.0)	8.37 (35.0)	4.16 (17.4)
Rye flour (whole grain)	3.05 (12.8)	8.37 (35.0)	3.86 (16.2)
Rye flour (light)	3.41 (14.3)	8.37 (35.0)	4.07 (17.0)
Sorghum (wholemeal)	0.91 (3.8)	8.37 (35.0)	4.03 (16.9)

Wheat (97 to 100 per cent extraction)	3.59 (14.0)	8.37 (35.0)	3.78 (15.8)
Wheat (70 to 74 per cent extraction)	4.05 (17.0)	8.37 (35.0)	4.12 (17.2)
Other cereals (refined)	3.87 (16.2)	8.37 (35.0)	4.12 (17.2)
Legumes, nuts:			
Mature dry beans, peas, nuts	3.47 (14.5)	8.37 (35.0)	4.07 (17.0)
Soybeans	3.47 (14.5)	8.37 (35.0)	4.07 (17.0)
Vegetables:			
Potatoes, starchy roots	2.78 (11.6)	8.37 (35.0)	4.03 (16.9)
Other underground crops	2.78 (11.6)	8.37 (35.0)	3.84 (16.1)
Other vegetables	2.44 (10.2)	8.37 (35.0)	3.57 (14.9)

Source:

Modified from Merrill AL & Watt BK (1973), 'Energy Value of Foods: Basis and Derivation', *Agriculture Handbook No. 74*, Washington, DC, ARS United States Department of Agriculture.

My calorie correction based on 'Net Metabolisable Energy'

9 calories per gram of **fat**
3.8 calories per gram of **sugar**
3.6 calories per gram of **complex carbs**
3.2 calories per gram of **protein**

So how does this work out in the real world? See below for the detailed calculations of the meal I described in Chapter 9. All nutritional and calorie values (aside from my corrections) come from the US Department of Agriculture (USDA) Agricultural Research Service 'Food Data Central' https://fdc.nal.usda.gov/

CAESAR SALAD (100G)

Energy	190kcal	Calculated from value per serving-size measure
Protein	5g	Calculated from value per serving-size measure
Total lipid (fat)	16g	Calculated from value per serving-size measure
Carbohydrate, by difference	8g	Calculated from value per serving-size measure
Fibre, total dietary	1g	Calculated from value per serving-size measure
Sugars, total including NLEA	2g	

The total **Atwater calorie-count** would be:

16g fat (16 × 9 = 144)

8g carbs (8 × 4 = 32)

5g protein (5 × 4 = 20)

Total = 144 + 32 + 20 = **196 calories**

My **NME correction** would be:

16g fat (16 × 9 = 144)

6g complex carbs (6 × 3.6 = 21.6)

2g sugars (2 × 3.8 = 7.6)

5 g protein (5 × 3.2 = 16)

Total = 144 + 21.6 + 7.6 + 16 = **189.2 calories**

RAW BEEF FILLET (200G)

11g of fat and 46g of protein.

The total **Atwater calorie-count** would be:

11g fat (11 × 9 = 99)

46g protein (46 × 4 = 184)

Total = 99 + 184 = **283 calories**

My **NME correction** would be:

11g fat (11 × 9 = 99)

 46g protein (46 × 3.2 calories = 147.2)

Total = 99 + 147.2 = **246.2 calories**

FRENCH FRIES (100G)

Energy	155kcal	Calculated from value per serving-size measure
Protein	2.38g	Calculated from value per serving-size measure
Total lipid (fat)	4.76g	Calculated from value per serving-size measure
Carbohydrate, by difference	25g	Calculated from value per serving-size measure
Fibre, total dietary	2.4g	Calculated from value per serving-size measure
Sugars, total including NLEA	1.19g	

The total **Atwater calorie-count** would be:

4.76g fat (4.76 × 9 = 42.84)

25g carbs (25 × 4 = 100)

2.38g protein (2.38 × 4 = 9.52)

Total = 42.84 + 100 + 9.52 = 152 calories; **200g portion = 304 calories**

My **NME correction** would be:

4.76g fat (4.76 × 9 = 42.84)

23.8g complex carbs (23.8 × 3.6 = 85.68)

1.2g sugars (1.2 × 3.8 = 4.56)

2.38g protein (2.38 × 3.2 = 7.6)

Total = 42.84 + 85.68 + 4.56 + 7.6 = 140.7 calories; **200g portion = 281.4 calories**

HORSERADISH SAUCE (100G)

Water	35.83g
Energy	503kcal
Protein	1.09g
Total lipid (fat)	50.89g
Carbohydrate, by difference	10.05g
Fibre, total dietary	1g
Sugars, total including NLEA	8.98g

The total **Atwater calorie-count** would be:

50.89g fat (50.89 × 9 = 458)

10.05g carbs (10.05 × 4 = 40.2)

1.09g protein (1.09 × 4 = 3.8)

Total = 458 + 40.2 + 3.8 = 502 calories; **25g portion = 125.5 calories**

My **NME correction** would be:

50.89g fat (50.89 × 9 = 458)

8.98g complex carbs (8.98 × 3.8 = 34.12)

1.07g sugars (1.07 × 3.6 = 3.9)

1.09g protein (1.09 × 3.2 = 3.5)

Total = 458 + 34.12 + 3.9 + 3.5 = 499.5 calories; **25g portion = 124.9 calories**

SLICE OF CHOCOLATE CAKE (100G)

16.67g of fat, 51.3g of carbs (37.2g from sugar, 14.1g from complex carbs), 3.85g of protein.

The total **Atwater calorie-count** would be:

16.67g fat (16.67 × 9 = 150)

51.3g carbs (51.3 × 4 = 205.2)

3.85g protein (3.85 × 4 = 15.4)

Total = 150 + 205.2 + 15.4 = **370.6 calories**

My **NME correction** would be:

16.67g fat (16.67 × 9 = 150)

14.1g complex carbs (14.1 × 3.6 = 50.76)

37.2g sugars (37.2 × 3.8 = 141.36)

3.85g protein (3.85 × 3.2 = 12.32)

Total = 150 + 50.76 + 141.36 + 12.32 = **354.4 calories**

That is 1280 total Atwater calories, which corrects to 1195 calories, a difference of 85 calories, or 6.6 per cent.

Recipes for some of my favourite 'no-rush' weekend dishes!

BEEF SHORT-RIB RENDANG

Rendang is a 'dry' Malaysian curry. When I say dry, there is a sauce, but it is very thick and clings to the meat. This works well with most cuts of stewing beef, lamb or chicken portions on the bone. Two important elements to this dish. The 'rempah' and slow cooking.

Rempah is the curry spice paste. You can actually buy this pre-made from good Asian or Chinese supermarkets, or even online. The only real difference in flavour in the homemade vs the pre-made pastes is that some of the 'volatiles' are missing and thus the finished product lacks just a touch of vibrancy. This can be fixed by throwing in some freshly chopped coriander and a squeeze of lime to the finished product.

Serves four, with steamed rice and a vegetable side dish, either steamed of stir-fried.

Ingredients

1.5kg beef short-rib

For the rempah:

5 dried red chillies

5 fresh chillies

1 thumb-sized piece galangal (otherwise known as 'Thai ginger' or 'blue ginger')

6 candlenuts (if you can't find these, use skinless almonds)

4 stalks fresh lemongrass, chopped

4 banana shallots or 2 medium onions

8 cloves garlic, peeled

100ml groundnut oil

1 tin coconut milk

1 tablespoon palm sugar (if you can't find this, use normal sugar)

2 teaspoons salt

230ml container worth grated coconut

300ml beef stock

Method

Put short-ribs fat side down into a dry frying pan on high heat. When you hear sizzling and see some fat rendering out, brown all sides of the ribs in their own fat for a few minutes, then take off the heat.

Place the chillies, galangal, candlenuts, lemongrass, shallots and garlic into a food processor and pulse until smooth. Loosen with a little water as required. Heat the oil in a heavy-bottom casserole dish. Add paste and stir until the paste incorporates with the oil. Turn down heat to medium and continue stirring until the rempah is fragrant, about 8 to 10 minutes. When the rempah begins to split and you can see red oil separating out, it is ready!

Add the beef ribs and coat in the rempah, then add the remaining ingredients, including the beef stock. Bring to boil, put the lid on, and place in a preheated oven at 160°C for at least three hours (no, you cannot shorten the process). At the two-hour mark, check to make sure the sauce hasn't become too dry. Add a little boiling water if necessary. Take the chance to skim off the fat that has gathered at the surface and discard. There will be quite a lot, so don't be scared! After three hours, thrown in a handful of freshly chopped coriander, a squeeze of lime, and enjoy with steamed rice!!

CHINESE BLACK BEEF BRISKET

Guys, don't be scared by the oodles of garlic in this dish. Once it's simmered for four hours, and you've incorporated it into the sauce, it becomes a mild sweet flavour full of umami goodness.

Serves 6 with steamed rice and a vegetable side dish, either steamed or stir-fried.

Ingredients

1.5kg beef brisket, either whole (from a butcher) or in two 700 to 800g joints. Available at most supermarkets.

3 tablespoons groundnut oil

250g garlic cloves, peeled (trust me)

3 tablespoons Shaoxing rice wine (if you can't find this, use medium-dry sherry)

1 teaspoon sugar

2 tablespoons dark soy sauce

1 tablespoon light soy sauce

500ml beef stock

1 tablespoon corn starch, dissolved in a little water

10 spring onions

Method

Heat oil in a heavy-bottom casserole dish. Brown all sides of the joint/s of beef. Add the whole garlic cloves and stir-fry until they pick up just a bit of colour. Splash in the rice wine, turn the beef in it, then add the soy sauces, sugar and stock. Bring to the boil, cover, and put into a preheated oven at 160°C for four hours (as above, no, you cannot shorten the process). At the two-hour and three-hour marks, turn the beef and check to make sure the sauce hasn't become too dry. Add a little boiling water if necessary.

After four hours, take out of the oven. Remove the beef from the sauce and put it somewhere warm to rest. Now to finish that killer sauce. Mash the soft garlic into the sauce, and place the casserole dish back on the heat. Add the corn starch and let the sauce thicken. Chop the spring onions into 3cm segments and add. Then, voila, the sauce is done! Taste and try not to faint at how divine it tastes . . . mmmm.

Now slice the beef, which, with all of that cooking, should be soft and melt-in-the-mouth unctuous. Pour the sauce over the slices of brisket and serve with steamed rice. Oy!

CRISPY AROMATIC DUCK WITH PANCAKES

And finally, this dish is what I call a low-effort high-impact dish! It makes you look like some uber-chef and is perfect for entertaining. There really isn't all that much meat on a duck, so if you can fit two ducks into the oven, then go nuts! Make sure you buy five spice with NO added salt or sugar. This allows you to control the seasoning.

Serves 6 as a starter or 3 as a main (because sometimes you need this for the whole meal).

Ingredients

One 1.2kg whole duck
5 tablespoons Chinese five spice
2 teaspoons salt
1 thumb-sized piece of root ginger

To serve:
10 spring onions
1 large cucumber
Hoisin sauce
Peking duck rice pancakes, available frozen from most Asian
    or Chinese supermarkets

Method

Pat dry the duck with a paper towel. Add the salt to the five-spice powder and mix. Grate the ginger and mix with 1 tablespoon of seasoned five spice. Then using your hand (no other way, chaps, roll your sleeves up) rub the inside of the duck with the grated ginger spice mixture. Rub the rest of the seasoned spice powder onto the whole duck. Place the duck on a rack within a roasting tray, which lets the fat drain off and gives you crispy skin, and into a preheated oven at 160°C for 1 hour 45 minutes.

Once the duck is cooked, put it somewhere warm to rest. Now prepare the accompaniments. Wrap as many pancakes as you would like into aluminium foil, and place in a steamer for 10 minutes. Cut the cucumber into 3cm × 0.5cm × 0.5cm bayonets. Slice the spring onions into 3cm segments, quarter them, and then pull them apart a bit more. Pour the hoisin sauce into a bowl with a teaspoon.

Now shred the rested duck with two forks.

Serve with a pancake, a little bit of hoisin sauce, a bit of duck, a bit of cucumber and spring onion. Roll up, and be prepared for flavour heaven. Oh, baby.

ACKNOWLEDGEMENTS

When I finished my PhD thesis, I thought 'Whew, that's that, I'm never going to write anything that long again!' Until, that was, I met my agent, Charlie, who somehow managed to winkle my first book out of me. Against all odds, lightning has apparently struck twice, and this is the result. So thank you so much, Charlie! I'd also like to thank Pippa and the entire team at Orion for believing in this project, and for continuing to provide me with a platform to speak loudly and fight stigma against those larger amongst us in society.

I am grateful to Dr Anna-Maria Siegert (Annemie), who works with me in Cambridge, and thoughtfully commented on early drafts (and incidentally speaks like five different languages). In particular, Annemie's help on distilling the key messages from the complexity of Chapter 3 was crucial. I'd also like to extend thanks to my colleague Prof. Alex Johnstone (University of Aberdeen) for lending her tremendous expertise on protein in diets and helping me out with Chapter 5.

Finally, the person I need to thank most is my wife, Jane, for her continued and unwavering support. Not only did Jane put up with me being ensconced in my office, as the book slowly emerged, throughout much of lockdown in the early part of 2020; she was (and continues to be) my 'muse', providing inspiration to multiple chapters, in addition to being responsible for most of the artwork in Chapter 3.

This book, as with much else in my life, is for Jane.

ABOUT THE AUTHOR

Giles Yeo is a geneticist with over 20 years' experience dedicated to researching obesity and the brain control of food intake. He obtained his PhD from the University of Cambridge and assisted the pioneering research that uncovered key pathways in how the brain controls food intake. His current research focuses on understanding how these pathways differ from person to person, and the influence of genetics in our relationship with food and eating habits. He is based at the MRC Metabolic Diseases Unit, where he is principal research associate, and is a fellow and graduate tutor at Wolfson College. Giles also moonlights as a science presenter for the BBC. In 2020, Giles was awarded an MBE in the Queen's Birthday Honours List for services to Research and Communication and Engagement.

He lives with his family in a little village with two windmills (one of which mills actual flour), two churches (one deconsecrated) and a pub, just outside Cambridge.

REFERENCES

1. Calories, calories everywhere

1. https://www.prevention.com/food-nutrition/a20457022/worst-foods-at-baseball-games/
2. https://www.nytimes.com/2020/02/02/us/politics/trump-kansas-city-chiefs-tweet.html
3. https://bleacherreport.com/articles/1812117-the-most-insanely-unhealthy-stadium-foods-ever-invented
4. https://www.food.gov.uk/business-guidance/nutrition-labelling
5. https://www.food.gov.uk/sites/default/files/media/document/fop-guidance_0.pdf
6. https://www.fda.gov/food/food-labeling-nutrition
7. https://www.food.gov.uk/sites/default/files/media/document/fop-guidance_0.pdf
8. https://www.fda.gov/food/food-labeling-nutrition/menu-labeling-requirements
9. https://www.gov.uk/government/news/public-health-responsibility-deal
10. https://www.telegraph.co.uk/news/2019/01/18/calorie-labels-will-placed-millions-takeaway-menus/
11. https://uk.deliveroo.news/news/calorie-labeling.html
12. https://www.telegraph.co.uk/news/2019/01/18/calorie-labels-will-placed-millions-takeaway-menus/
13. https://uk.deliveroo.news/news/calorie-labeling.html
14. https://www.acs.org/content/acs/en/education/whatischemistry/landmarks/lavoisier.html
15. Lavoisier, Antoine (1790), *Elements of Chemistry in New Systematic Order, Containing All Modern Discoveries, Illustrated with Thirteen Copperplates,* translated from the French by Robert Kerr (1st ed.).
16. Buchholz AC and Schoeller DA (2004), 'Is a calorie a calorie?', *American Journal of Clinical Nutrition* vol. 79 (suppl), pp.899S–906S.
17. https://www.acs.org/content/acs/en/education/whatischemistry/landmarks/lavoisier.html
18. Hargrove JL (2006), 'History of the Calorie in Nutrition', *The Journal of Nutrition* vol. 136, pp.2957–2961.

2. The Atwater factor

1. 'Obituary of Max Rubner', *Nature*, 3268, vol. 129, p.893, 1932.
2. Treitel, C (2008), 'Max Rubner and the Biopolitics of Rational Nutrition', *Central European History*, vol. 41, pp.1–25.
3. Hargrove, JL (2006), 'History of the Calorie', *Nutrition. J. Nutr.* vol. 136, pp.2957–2961.
4. True, AC (1908), 'Wilbur Olin Atwater 1844–1907', *Proceedings of the Washington Academy of Sciences*, vol. 10, pp.194–198.
5. Widdowson, EM (1955), 'Assessment of the Energy Value of Foods', *Proceedings of the Nutritional Society*, vol. 4, pp.142–54.
6. Widdowson EM (1987), 'Atwater: A Personal Tribute from the United Kingdom', *American Journal Clinical Nutrition*, vol. 45, pp.898–904.
7. Atwater WO & Woods CD (1896), 'The Chemical Composition of American Food Materials', Washington, DC: US Government Printing Office. *US Dept of Agriculture Office of Experiment Stations, Bulletin no. 28.*
8. Atwater WO (1902), *Principles of Nutrition and Nutritive Value of Food*, Washington, DC: US Government Printing Office. Corrected 1910; reprinted 1916. *US Dept of Agriculture Office of Experiment Stations, Bulletin no. 142.*
9. Widdowson EM (1955), 'Assessment of the Energy Value of Foods', *Proceedings of the Nutritional Society*, vol. 4, pp.142–54.
10. Atwater WO & Bryant AP (1900), 'The Availability and Fuel Values of Food Materials', Connecticut (Storrs) Agricultural Experiment Station 12th Annual Report, 1899.
11. Atwater WO & Bryant AP (1900), 'The Availability and Fuel Values of Food Materials', Connecticut (Storrs) Agricultural Experiment Station 12th Annual Report, 1899.
12. Atwater WO (1902), *Principles of Nutrition and Nutritive Value of Food*, Washington, DC: US Government Printing Office. Corrected 1910; reprinted 1916. *US Dept of Agriculture Office of Experiment Stations, Bulletin no. 142.*
13. Atwater WO, Rosa EB (1899), 'Description of a New Respiration Calorimeter and Experiments on the Conservation Energy in the Human Body', Washington, DC: US Government Printing Office. *US Department of Agriculture Office of Experiment Stations, Bulletin no. 63.*
14. Atwater WO, Benedict FG (1899), 'Experiments on the Metabolism of Matter and Energy in the Human Body', Washington, DC: US Government Printing Office. *US Department of Agriculture Office of Experiment Stations, Bulletin no. 69.*
15. Atwater WO (1903), 'The Nutritive Value of Alcohol' in *Physiological Aspects of the Liquor Problem*, vol. 2. Boston, MA, and New York, NY: Houghton, Mifflin and Co, pp.174–347.
16. Atwater WO, Benedict FG (1902), 'Experiments on the Metabolism of Matter and Energy in the Human Body, 1898–1900', Washington, DC: US Government Printing Office. *US Department of Agriculture Office of Experiment Stations, Bulletin no. 109.*
17. Peters LH (1918), *Diet and Health with Key to the Calories*, Chicago: Reilly and Lee.
18. Peters LH (1918), *Diet and Health with Key to the Calories*, Chicago: Reilly and Lee.
19. https://www.npr.org/2014/08/05/337860700/bra-history-how-a-war-shortage-reshaped-modern-shapewear?t=1594914200236

20. https://www.ocf.berkeley.edu/~immer/books1920s
21. Atwater WO (1902), *Principles of Nutrition and Nutritive Value of Food*, Washington, DC: US Government Printing Office. Corrected 1910; reprinted 1916. *US Dept of Agriculture Office of Experiment Stations, Bulletin no. 142.*
22. Jones DB (1931), 'Factors for Converting Percentages of Nitrogen in Foods and Feeds into Percentages of Protein', *USDA* (US Department of Agriculture) *Circular Series*, No. 183, pp.1–21.
23. Merrill AL, Watt BK (1955), 'Energy Value of Foods-Basis and Derivation', Washington, DC: US Government Printing Office. *US Department of Agriculture Handbook no. 74.*

3. How do we turn food into energy?

1. Itan, Y, Powell, A, Beaumont, MA, Burger, J & Thomas, MG (2009), 'The Origins of Lactase Persistence in Europe', *PLOS Computational Biology* vol. 5, e1000491, doi:10.1371/journal.pcbi.1000491.
2. https://www.nobelprize.org/prizes/medicine/1953/summary/
3. https://www.nobelprize.org/prizes/chemistry/1978/summary/
4. https://www.nobelprize.org/prizes/chemistry/1997/summary/
5. Bliss, Michael (1982), *The Discovery of Insulin*, Chicago, The University of Chicago Press.
6. https://www.nobelprize.org/prizes/medicine/1923/summary/

4. What do we use energy for?

1. Rubner M (1883), 'Zeitschrift fur Biologie' vol. 19, pp.536–562.
2. Kleiber M (1932), 'Body size and metabolism' *Hilgardia* vol. 6, pp.315–353.
3. Atwater WO, Rosa EB, (1899), 'Description of a New Respiration Calorimeter and Experiments on the Conservation Energy in the Human Body' Washington, DC: Government Printing Office; *US Department of Agriculture Office of Experiment Stations, Bulletin 63.*

5. The power of protein

1. Murphy KG, Dhillo WS, and Bloom SR (2006), 'Gut Peptides in the Regulation of Food Intake and Energy Homeostasis', *Endocrine Reviews*, vol. 27(7), pp. 719–727.
2. Cummings DE, Rubino F (Feb 2018), 'Metabolic Surgery for the Treatment of Type 2 Diabetes in Obese Individuals', *Diabetologia*, vol. 61(2), pp. 257–264. doi: 10.1007/s00125-017-4513-y. Epub 2017 Dec 9. Review. PMID: 29224190.
3. Manning S, Pucci A, Batterham RL (Mar 2015) 'Roux-en-Y Gastric Bypass: Effects on Feeding Behavior and Underlying Mechanisms', *Journal of Clinical Investigation*, vol. 2;125(3): pp.939–48. doi: 10.1172/JCI76305. Epub 2015 Mar 2. Review. PMID: 25729850.
4. Chakravartty S, Tassinari D, Salerno A, Giorgakis E, Rubino F (Jun 2015), 'What is the Mechanism Behind Weight Loss Maintenance with Gastric Bypass?', *Current Obesity Reports*, vol. 4(2), pp.262–8. doi: 10.1007/s13679-015-0158-7. Review. PMID: 26627220.

5. Behary P, Tharakan G, Alexiadou K, Johnson N, Wewer Albrechtsen NJ, Kenkre J, Cuenco J, Hope D, Anyiam O, Choudhury S, Alessimii H, Poddar A, Minnion J, Doyle C, Frost G, Le Roux C, Purkayastha S, Moorthy K, Dhillo W, Holst JJ, Ahmed AR, Prevost AT, Bloom SR, Tan TM (Aug 2019), 'Combined GLP-1, Oxyntomodulin, and Peptide YY Improves Body Weight and Glycemia in Obesity and Prediabetes/Type 2 Diabetes: A Randomized, Single-Blinded, Placebo-Controlled Study', *Diabetes Care*, vol. 42(8), pp.1446–1453. doi: 10.2337/dc19-0449. Epub 2019 Jun 8.PMID: 31177183.

6. Johnstone, A (2013), 'Protein and Satiety' in J. Blundell, & F. Bellisle (eds.), *Satiation, Satiety and the Control of Food Intake: Theory and Practice* (pp. 128–142), Woodhead Publishing Series in Food Science, Technology and Nutrition, Woodhead Publishing.

7. Neacsu M, Fyfe C, Horgan G, and Johnstone AM (2014), 'Appetite Control and Biomarkers of Satiety with Vegetarian (Soy) and Meat-based High-protein Diets for Weight Loss in Obese Men: A Randomized Crossover Trial', *American Journal Clinical Nutrition*, vol. 100, pp.548–58.

8. Halton TL, Hu FB (Oct 2004), 'The Effects of High Protein Diets on Thermogenesis, Satiety and Weight Loss: A Critical Review', *Journal of the American College of Nutrition* vol. 23(5), pp.373–85.

9. Atkins RC, *Dr. Atkins' Diet Revolution*, Bantam Books (first published Jan 1, 1972).

10. Banting W (1864) 'Letter on Corpulence: Addressed to the Public', New York.

11. https://www.huffingtonpost.co.uk/2017/04/21/tim-noakes-found-not-guilty-of-misconduct-over-advising-mother-t_a_22049207/

12. https://uk.atkins.com/

13. http://www.dukandiet.co.uk/

14. https://www.mayoclinic.org/healthy-lifestyle/weight-loss/in-depth/south-beach-diet/art-20048491

15. Wilder RM, (1921), 'The Effect of Ketonemia on the Course of Epilepsy', *Mayo Clinic Bulletin* 2, p.307.

16. Shimazu T, Hirschey MD, Newman J, He W, Shirakawa K, Le Moan N, Grueter CA, Lim H, Saunders LR, Stevens RD, Newgard CB, Farese Jr RV, de Cabo R, Ulrich S, Akassoglou K, Verdin E (Jan 2013), 'Suppression of Oxidative Stress by β-hydroxybutyrate, an Endogenous Histone Deacetylase Inhibitor', *Science*, vol. 339(6116), pp.211–4.

17. https://www.menshealth.com/nutrition/a25775330/keto-diet-history/

18. Yeo G (2018), *Gene Eating: The Story of Human Appetite*, Orion Publishing Group, chapter 5.

19. Cordain L (2001), *The Paleo Diet: Lose Weight and Get Healthy by Eating the Foods You Were Designed to Eat*, John Wiley & Sons.

20. Baker S (2018), *The Carnivore Diet*, Victory Belt Publishing.

21. Ebbeling CB, Feldman HA, Klein GL, Wong JMW, Bielak L, Steltz SK, Luoto PK, Wolfe RR, Wong WW, Ludwig DS (2018), 'Effects of a Low Carbohydrate Diet on Energy Expenditure During Weight Loss Maintenance: Randomized Trial', *BMJ*, vol. 363, k4583.

6. The wonder of fibre

1. Burkitt DP (1969), 'Related Disease – Related Cause', *Lancet*, vol. ii, pp.1229–1231.
2. Burkitt DP & O'Conor GT (1961), 'Malignant Lymphoma in African Children. I. A Clinical Syndrome', *Cancer*, vol. 14, pp.258–269.
3. Painter NS (1967), 'Diet and Diverticulosis' *BMJ* 3, p.434.
4. Walker ARP, Walker BF & Richardson BD (1970), 'Bowel Transit Times in Bantu Populations', *BMJ*, vol. 3, pp.48–49.
5. Cleave TL & Campbell GD (1966), *Diabetes, Coronary Thrombosis and the Saccharine Disease*, Bristol: John Wright and Sons.
6. Cummings JH and Engineer A (2018), 'Denis Burkitt and the Origins of the Dietary Fibre Hypothesis', *Nutrition Research Reviews*, vol. 31, pp.1–15.
7. Burkitt DP (1969), 'Related Disease – Related Cause', *Lancet*, vol. ii, pp.1229–1231.
8. Burkitt DP (1970), 'Relationship as a Clue to Causation' *Lancet*, vol. ii, pp.1237–1240.
9. O'Keefe SJ (2019), 'The Association Between Dietary Fibre Deficiency and High Income Lifestyle-Associated Diseases: Burkitt's Hypothesis Revisited', *Lancet* Gastroenterology and Hepatology, vol. 4(12), pp.984–996.
10. Bingham SA, Day NE, Luben R, et al. (2003), 'Dietary Fibre in Food and Protection Against Colorectal Cancer in the European Prospective Investigation into Cancer and Nutrition (EPIC): an Observational Study', *Lancet*, vol. 361, pp.1496–501.
11. Reynolds A, Mann J, Cummings J, Winter N, Mete E, Te Morenga L (2019), 'Carbohydrate Quality and Human Health: a Series of Systematic Reviews and Meta-Analyses', *Lancet*, vol. 393, pp.434–5.
12. Yu EW, Gao L, Stastka P, Cheney MC, Mahabamunuge J, Torres Soto M, et al. (2020), 'Fecal Microbiota Transplantation for the Improvement of Metabolism in Obesity: The FMTTRIM Double-Blind Placebo-Controlled Pilot Trial', *PLOS Med*, vol. 17(3): e1003051.
13. Byrne CS, Chambers ES, Morrisonm DJ and Frost G (2015), 'The Role of Short Chain Fatty Acids in Appetite Regulation and Energy Homeostasis', *International Journal of Obesity*, vol. 39, pp.1331–1338.
14. Chambers ES, Preston T, Frost G & Morrison DJ (2018), 'Role of Gut Microbiota-Generated Short-Chain Fatty Acids in Metabolic and Cardiovascular Health', *Current Nutrition Reports*, vol. 7, pp.198–206
15. Cummings JH and Engineer A (2018), 'Denis Burkitt and the Origins of the Dietary Fibre Hypothesis', *Nutrition Research Reviews*, vol. 31, pp.1–15.
16. Crapo PA, Reaven G & Olefsky J (1976), 'Plasma Glucose and Insulin Responses to Orally Administered Simple and Complex Carbohydrates', *Diabetes*, vol. 25, pp.741–747.
17. Jenkins DJA, Wolever TMS, Taylor RH, et al. (1981), 'Glycemic Index of Foods: a Physiological Basis for Carbohydrate Exchange', *American Journal of Clinical Nutrition*, vol. 34, pp.362–366.
18. https://yougov.co.uk/topics/consumer/articles-reports/2011/09/23/love-it-hate-it-its-official
19. Estruch R, Ros E, Jordi Salas-Salvadó J, Covas M, Corella D, Arós F, Gómez-Gracia E, Ruiz-Gutiérrez V, Fiol M, Lapetra J, Lamuela-Raventos RM, Serra-Majem L, et al., for the PREDIMED Study Investigators (2018), 'Primary Prevention of Cardiovascular Disease with a Mediterranean Diet Supplemented with Extra-Virgin Olive Oil or Nuts', *New England Journal Medicine*, vol. 378, e34.

20. https://www.who.int/health-topics/cardiovascular-diseases#tab=tab_1
21. https://www.insider.com/daniel-diet-sirtfood-weird-celebrity-diets-2019-6
22. http://www.thesirtfooddiet.com/
23. Goggins A & Matten G (2016), *The Sirtfood Diet*, Hodder & Stoughton
24. Young RO and Young SR (2003), *The pH Miracle: Balance your Diet, Reclaim your Health*, Warner Books, paperback edition
25. https://www.vox.com/2019/1/30/18203676/tom-brady-diet-book-water

7. The 'ultra' in processed

1. Monteiro CA (2009), 'Nutrition and Health. The issue is not food, nor nutrients, so much as processing', *Public Health Nutrition*, vol. 12(5), pp.729–731.
2. Monteiro CA, Cannon G, Levy RB *et al.* (2016), '*NOVA*. The star shines bright' *[Food classification. Public health] World Nutrition*, vol. 7, pp.1–3, 28–38
3. Monteiro CA (2009), 'Nutrition and health. The issue is not food, nor nutrients, so much as processing', *Public Health Nutrition*, vol. 12(5), pp.729–731.
4. Vandevijvere S, Jaacks LM, Monteiro CA, Moubarac J, Girling-Butcher M, Lee AC, Pan A, Bentham J & Swinburn B (2019), 'Global Trends in Ultraprocessed Food and Drink Product Sales and their Association with Adult Body Mass Index Trajectories', *Obesity Reviews*, vol. 10;20(S2), pp.10–19. Supplementary Material 1.
5. Martines RM, Machado PP, Neri DA, Levy RB, Rauber F (2019), 'Association Between Watching TV Whilst Eating and Children's Consumption of Ultraprocessed Foods in United Kingdom', *Maternal and Child Nutrition*, vol. 15(4): e12819.
6. Vandevijvere S, Jaacks LM, Monteiro CA, Moubarac J, Girling-Butcher M, Lee AC, Pan A, Bentham J & Swinburn B (2019), 'Global Trends in Ultraprocessed Food and Drink Product Sales and their Association With Adult Body Mass Index Trajectories', *Obesity Reviews*, vol. 10;20(S2), pp.10–19. Supplementary Material 1.
7. Monteiro CA, Moubarac JC, Levy RB, Canella DS, Louzada MLDC, Cannon G (2018), 'Household Availability of Ultra-processed Foods and Obesity in Nineteen European Countries', *Public Health Nutrition*, vol. 21(1), pp.18–26.
8. Pan American Health Organization, 'Ultra-processed food and drink products in Latin America: trends, impact on obesity, policy implications', Washington D.C: Pan American Health Organization; 2015.
9. Vandevijvere S, Jaacks LM, Monteiro CA, Moubarac J, Girling-Butcher M, Lee AC, Pan A, Bentham J & Swinburn B (2019), 'Global Trends in Ultraprocessed Food and Drink Product Sales and their Association With Adult Body Mass Index Trajectories', *Obesity Reviews*, vol. 10;20(S2), pp.10–19.
10. Barr SB and Wright JC (2010), 'Postprandial Energy Expenditure in Whole-food and Processed-food Meals: Implications for Daily Energy Expenditure', *Food & Nutrition Research*, vol. 54, p.5144.
11. Hall KD, Ayuketah A, Brychta R, Cai H et al. (2019), 'Ultra-Processed Diets Cause Excess Calorie Intake and Weight Gain: An Inpatient Randomized Controlled Trial of Ad Libitum Food Intake', *Cell Metabolism*, vol. 30, pp.1–11.
12. Simpson SJ, Raubenheimer D (2005), 'Obesity: The Protein Leverage Hypothesis', *Obesity Review*, vol. 6(2), pp.133–42.
13. DiFeliceantonio AG, Coppin G, Rigoux L, Thanarajah SE, Dagher A, Tittgemeyer M and Small DM (2018), 'Supra-Additive Effects of Combining Fat and Carbohydrate

on Food Reward', *Cell Metabolism*, vol. 28, pp.33–44.

14. https://www.vice.com/en_uk/article/9kpdqa/the-uks-first-vegan-cheese-shop-isnt-afraid-of-controversy

15. https://www.sfgate.com/food/article/Plant-based-burger-battle-heats-up-as-Impossible-13596414.php?t=0383071c06&ipid=sfgatehp

16. https://medium.com/impossible-foods/heme-health-the-essentials-95201e5afffa

17. https://www.sfgate.com/food/article/Plant-based-burger-battle-heats-up-as-Impossible-13596414.php?t=0383071c06&ipid=sfgatehp

18. https://nypost.com/2019/06/08/brooklyn-burger-king-caught-replacing-meatless-impossible-whoppers-with-beef/

19. Monteiro CA, Cannon G, Moubarac J, Levy RB, Louzada MLC and Jaime PC (2017), 'The UN Decade of Nutrition, the NOVA Food Classification and the Trouble with Ultra-processing', *Public Health Nutrition*, vol. 21(1), pp.5–17.

20. Monteiro CA, Cannon G, Moubarac J, Levy RB, Louzada MLC and Jaime PC (2017), 'The UN Decade of Nutrition, the NOVA Food Classification and the Trouble with Ultra-processing', *Public Health Nutrition*, vol. 21(1), pp.5–17.

8. Privilege and calories

1. http://www.fao.org/in-action/voices-of-the-hungry/fies/en/

2. https://publications.parliament.uk/pa/cm201719/cmselect/cmenvaud/1491/149105.htm#footnote-189-backlink

3. https://www.ers.usda.gov/topics/food-nutrition-assistance/food-security-in-the-us/key-statistics-graphics.aspx

4. https://www.bbc.co.uk/news/education-49515117

5. https://foodfoundation.org.uk/vulnerable_groups/new-poll-data-more-than-five-million-people-in-households-with-children-have-experienced-food-insecurity-since-lockdown-began/

6. Stunkard AJ, Foch TT, Hrubec Z (1986), 'A Twin Study of Human Obesity', *JAMA*, vol. 256, pp.51–54.

7. Stunkard AJ, Harris JR, Pedersen NL, McClearn GE (1990), 'The Body-mass Index of Twins who have been Reared Apart', *New England Journal of Medicine*, vol. 322, pp.1483–1487.

8. van Jaarsveld CHM, Johnson L, Llewellyn C, Wardle J (2010), 'Gemini: a UK Twin Birth Cohort with a Focus on Early Childhood Weight Trajectories, Appetite and the Family Environment', *Twin Research Human Genetics*, vol. 13(1), pp.72–78.

9. Schrempft S, van Jaarsveld CHM, Fisher A, Herle M, Smith AD, Fildes A, Llewellyn CH (2018), 'Variation in the Heritability of Child Body Mass Index by Obesogenic Home Environment', *JAMA Pediatr.*, vol. 172(12), pp.1153–1160.

10. Marmot M, Allen J, Boyce T, Goldblatt P, Morrison J. (2020), 'Health equity in England: The Marmot Review 10 years on'. London: Institute of Health Equity

11. 'The State of the World's Children 2019 Executive Summary. Children, Food and Nutrition: Growing Well in a Changing World', published by the United Nations Children's Fund (UNICEF) October 2019.

12. https://www.hsj.co.uk/comment/the-bedpan-the-poor-cant-afford-to-follow-public-health-advice/7025532.article

13. Hall KD, Ayuketah A, Brychta R, Cai H et al. (2019), 'Ultra-Processed Diets Cause

Excess Calorie Intake and Weight Gain: An Inpatient Randomized Controlled Trial of Ad Libitum Food Intake', *Cell Metabolism*, vol. 30, pp.1–11.

14. Maguire ER, Burgoine T, Monsivais P (2015), 'Area Deprivation and the Food Environment Over Time: A Repeated Cross-sectional Study on Takeaway Outlet Density and Supermarket Presence in Norfolk, UK, 1990–2008', *Health & Place*, vol. 33, pp.142–147.

15. https://publications.parliament.uk/pa/cm201719/cmselect/cmhealth/882/88209. htm

9. We don't eat calories, we eat food

1. Vidal-Puig A (2013), 'Adipose Tissue Expandability, Lipotoxicity and the Metabolic Syndrome', *Endocrinol Nutrition*, 201360 Suppl. 1, pp.39–43.

2. Lotta LA, Gulati P, Day FR, Payne F, et al. (2017), 'Integrative Genomic Analysis Implicates Limited Peripheral Adipose Storage Capacity in the Pathogenesis of Human Insulin Resistance', *Nature Genetics*, vol. 49(1), pp.17–26.

3. Crockett RA, King SE, Marteau TM, Prevost AT, Bignardi G, Roberts NW, Stubbs B, Hollands GJ, Jebb SA (2018), 'Nutritional Labelling for Healthier Food or Non-alcoholic Drink Purchasing and Consumption', *Cochrane Database Syst Rev.* 27;2:CD009315.

4. Swift DL, Johannsen NM, Lavie CJ, Earnest CP & Church TS (2014), 'The Role of Exercise and Physical Activity in Weight Loss and Maintenance', *Progress in Cardiovascular Diseases*, vol. 56, pp.441–447.

5. King NA, Hopkins M, Caudwell P, Stubbs RJ & Blundell JE (2009), 'Beneficial Effects of Exercise: Shifting the Focus From Body Weight to Other Markers of Health', *British Journal of Sports Medicine*, vol. 43, pp.924–927.

6. Merrill AL, Watt BK (1955), 'Energy Value of Foods-basis and Derivation', Washington, DC: US Government Printing Office. *US Dept Agriculture Handbook* no. 74.

7. Livesey G (2001), 'A Perspective on Food Energy Standards for Nutrition Labelling', *British Journal of Nutrition*, vol. 85, pp.271–287.

INDEX